The Note on the Mirror

The Note
on the
Mirror

*Pregnant Teenagers
Tell Their Stories*

Julia C. Loren

Zondervan Publishing House
Grand Rapids, Michigan

The Note on the Mirror
Pregnant Teenagers Tell Their Stories

Copyright © 1990 by Julia C. Loren
All rights reserved

Published by Zondervan Publishing House
1415 Lake Drive, S.E., Grand Rapids, Michigan 49506

Library of Congress Cataloging-in-Publication Data

Loren, Julia C.
    The note on the mirror : pregnant teenagers tell their stories /
Julia C. Loren
        p. cm.
    "Youth books."
    ISBN 0-310-53531-X
    1. Teenage mothers—United States. 2. Teenage pregnancy—United
States. 3. Adoption—United States. 4. Abortion—United States.
I. Title.
HQ759.4.L67   1990
306.85'6—dc20   90–40833
                                                           CIP

Printed in the United States of America

90 91 92 93 94 / LP / 10 9 8 7 6 5 4 3 2 1

In memory of Jim Myers

CONTENTS

Acknowledgments

To the eight women whose stories and tears fill the following pages:

Thank you for your courage in sharing your story, your openness in revealing your pain, and your love that dances so freely upon these pages.

A Message to the Reader

I don't know about you, but life doesn't always turn out the way I'd planned. In fact, life tends to stick its giant foot out and trip me up on a daily basis. Either that or it purposely kicks me in the you-know-what.

When I was in high school, I didn't realize that this foot was following me everywhere I went, ready to stamp out my dreams. At sixteen I dreamed of traveling around the world, of going to college, of writing poems and stories. I figured that someday I would settle down, get married, and maybe have children.

My plans were good, but my life at sixteen years of age was a different story. It consisted of high school parties, competing in swimming and diving, heartbreaks caused by boyfriends, and arguments with family members and close girlfriends. Schoolwork came second to parties and pleasure. I didn't take life seriously. My work consisted of building castles in the air.

But all that changed seemingly overnight. I became pregnant. And my life changed drastically.

What do I do now? I wondered. For months I agonized over my dilemma. When I finally told my parents, they said they would support me in whatever decision I made. All I had to do was decide what I wanted to do. But I didn't even know what my options were.

When I told my boyfriend Paul, he said he would pay for an abortion. A couple of days later, he changed his mind and said he wanted me to have the child and move in with him. Then he offered to marry me, as if that would cement our relationship. Finally, he realized that I didn't want to settle into family life with him and threatened to take me to court and sue me for custody of the baby. I couldn't believe this soap opera situation was happening to me. This wasn't me. This wasn't my life.

But it *was* my life. With each passing month, that fact grew harder to deny. I needed to make some tough decisions—soon.

Unlike many parents, my parents didn't tell me what to do with the baby but let me struggle with the decision myself. I procrastinated so long in making a decision that it grew too late for an abortion. But I didn't really mind, for I thought of abortion as an easy way to cover the fact that I had sex with my boyfriend and "got caught." Besides, I was influenced by one of my favorite TV shows at the time, "Baretta." The star of the show, a dumpy cop with a pet parrot, always said, "Don't do the crime if you can't pay the time." He repeated it so often that he began to sound like a parrot himself. Nevertheless, the phrase stuck in my mind. And I decided to pay the time.

After six months of pregnancy, I still had no idea what I was going to do with a child. A baby just didn't fit into my plans. How could I travel in Europe and go to college if I had a baby? This pregnancy disrupted everything.

Slowly it dawned on me that I had someone else's life to consider. My life wasn't my own anymore. Someone was growing inside of me. The decisions I faced were going to determine the life of the child growing inside of me as well as my own. I became very serious. And I became seriously depressed as I tried to figure out what to do.

At age seventeen, at the end of my senior year of high school, I gave birth to a little girl. Then I gave her to another couple for adoption. I knew I wasn't ready for parenthood and thought they could raise her better than I could at the time.

Today, I know I was right in making that decision.

However, it took many years before I could feel good about having given up a part of my life to total strangers. But I know that the decision I made then was the best decision under the circumstances. And I know that another Being carefully guided me in the decision-making process and directed the outcome of many lives. The gentle hand of God was leading me all along.

I know that many of you who read this book may never become pregnant. My hope for you is that the stories contained in this book will lodge in your heart and mind and that you will avoid the pain of unplanned pregnancy.

If you are reading this book because you are pregnant, you are probably facing many of the same decisions I dealt with in high school. Questions bombard you daily. Who do I tell? What do I do? You feel overwhelmed, frightened, angry. Most of all, you feel alone. Your boyfriend may have been there to get you pregnant, but he's no better equipped than you to know what to do with a baby. So where do you turn?

This book is here to tell you: You are not alone. You are not the only one who ever found herself pregnant and confused about what to do. Every young woman I interviewed in this book found herself in your situation. As you read their stories, take note of how they decided what to do with an unplanned pregnancy. Maybe they will help you find what direction to take as you consider your options.

Before you read, take a moment to ask God to guide you in making the decision that is right for your life and the life of your child. Try this for starters, "God, help!" In a crisis state of mind, you may find yourself unable to say more. But if you have calmed down enough to pray longer, ask God for direction, for courage, for support.

You are not alone. God is with you. Whether or not you believe in God, now is the time to discover that he really does care about you and is even now standing by your side waiting for you to talk to him about all your confusion. I promise, you'll feel a lot more peaceful once you start talking.

In this book I have chosen to limit myself to the topic of unplanned pregnancy and deciding between the options: adoption, abortion, or parenting. It is impossible to cover all of the related topics surrounding sex and pregnancy; therefore I do not discuss sexually transmitted diseases or contraceptives and how to obtain them. If you have questions about these or other issues, I encourage you to talk with someone you trust or to call one of the telephone numbers listed in this book.

Don't be afraid to ask someone about birth control. It's better to be prepared, even if you're not planning to have sex. Some of the girls mentioned in the following stories didn't plan for sex; it "just happened." If they had considered what could "just happen," maybe they would have abstained that night and resisted the temptations. Or maybe they would have been prepared to prevent pregnancy from occurring. Just one sexual encounter is enough to get pregnant or contract herpes or AIDS. That one encounter can alter your life forever.

If you are not prepared to find out about birth control on your own, you are not ready for sex. Even more to the point: If you are not prepared to raise a child, you are not ready for sex. You may be mature enough to use birth control, but are you equipped to raise a baby in the event that the birth control fails? I wasn't. Neither were any of the girls I interviewed.

Read on.

Maybe you will find your story in the pages to follow.

PART I
Adoption

The Adoption Option

"I could never do what you did. How could you ever give your baby away?"

"Why did you go through nine months of pregnancy when you could have gotten an abortion?"

When at age seventeen I released my baby for adoption, I heard many callous words like these. But I knew that these people hadn't gone through what I'd gone through. They had no understanding of what adoption is all about. Releasing your child for adoption isn't selfish, as the first speaker implies. Nor is it stupid to have your baby, as the other person claims.

The girls in this first section of the book also faced doubts and opposition when they decided to release their child. But each one feels it was the best decision she could have made. Before we read their stories, however, let's take a look at what adoption is, the effects of adoption, and the kinds of adoption available.

THE IDEAL MOM

Picture the ideal mother. Perhaps she is a friend's mother, or someone on television you admire. What do you like about her? How does she relate to her children? How old was she when she started having children and raising a family?

Now, put yourself in the place of your ideal mother. Are you a lot like her? Do you think you could be the same kind of mother with the same degree of maturity as your ideal mom? These are heavy questions, but I have one more question for you.

Would you want your baby to be raised by a mom like you or a mom like her?

Most girls who release a child for adoption do so because they decide that another family could give the best care to their child. They recognize that raising a baby takes more than they have to give—emotionally, financially, physically, materially, and spiritually. They are not ready to be moms. And their boyfriends are not ready to be dads. Some girls decide that their baby would be better off in a family that has both a mother and a father.

That is what adoption is all about: giving your child an opportunity to be loved and nurtured by someone who is ready to make that sacrifice. Adoption is choosing to let go of the baby, allowing someone else to love it no matter how badly you desire to love the child or have the child love you.

THE EFFECTS OF ADOPTION

Today, despite the comments of others, adoption is more acceptable. But due to the availability of abortions, fewer infants find their way into loving families. Pregnant girls from affluent areas are more likely to seek abortions. Minority teens have a higher rate of teen births and tend to keep their children. Most pregnant teens drop out of high school. Very few attend college. It's hard to be poor and raise a child.

But it's hard to release a child for adoption, too. Not only do you have to release the child; so does your boyfriend, the grandparents, and your whole family.

However, you bear the brunt of the decision. The effects on you, the mother, are going to be the most difficult. When you first decide to release your child for adoption, you will feel an initial sense of relief. But making a decision won't stop the doubts you have. Even after the baby is born and placed in another home, you will wonder if what you did was right. Sensing your loss, you will grieve.

It takes some young women a long time to get over their loss, but it doesn't have to. Those women who decide on adoption early in the pregnancy and who have supportive friends will have an easier time. Those friends are still important later in life, on the child's birthday, for instance, when the birth mother will wonder what her child's life is like. At such times birth mothers will need someone to talk to. Adoption is an ongoing process that takes years to work through. Any teenage pregnancy, no matter what decision is made, is going to affect the girl for years to come.

Happily, adoption has more positive than negative side effects. A young woman who releases her child for adoption can move on with her own life, knowing that the baby is being loved and cared for. She doesn't have to struggle with finances, or cancel dates to care for her child. Instead, she can take charge of her life, dealing with her own problems before she takes on the responsibilities of another's life.

What about the effects on the baby? Child development experts say that the first five years of the baby's life are the formative years, setting the stage for how the child will respond to life. When I was wondering about adoption, I heard this and decided that it would take at least five years for me to get my act together and grow up enough to take care of a child. How would I affect my child during those five years? I saw myself struggling to become a person with enough ability to train up a child. I didn't want to be a tired out single mom, frustrated over not having enough money to pay bills and yelling at the baby to shut up so I could get some sleep.

Only you know how prepared you are to be a mother. I have met a couple of teenage mothers who were great

The Adoption Option

moms. But they had a lot of help from their own families and people in their churches. And it still was very difficult.

There are lots of other pros and cons about adoption. As you read the stories of the girls in this section you'll be able to spot the areas of joy and the areas of difficulty that come with making the decision to adopt.

What you won't see, however, are the different kinds of adoption available today. Birth mothers have a great deal of control over what kind of home they are able to choose for their child, whether or not they want to have any contact with the child, and who is to be involved in the adoption process. Birth fathers have few rights in the decision-making process. However, in the future, birth fathers may be given more legal say over the destiny of their unborn child. They will have to be included in the decision.

Adopting couples usually have to wait for years to adopt a child, for there simply aren't enough children available for adoption partially due to the number of women who choose to have abortions. Every child is a wanted child. If you decide to release your child for adoption, you can be sure that your child will be dearly loved by its adoptive parents.

TYPES OF ADOPTION

Here are the types of adoption available. If you decide you want further information on adoption, look into the chapter titled "Adoption: Step-by-Step."

Private Adoption

Private adoptions are arranged through attorneys, who act as a liaison between the birth mother and adopting couple and who take care of all the legal work. The attorney should be able to list a variety of prospective families who want to adopt and answer any questions you may have about these couples. In turn, the attorney will ask you to provide information about you and the baby's father, which the attorney will present to the adopting couple. The attorney may also arrange for you to meet the couple if you want to, or work out a plan for you to have contact with your child after it is born, either through letters or visits. This is called "Open Adoption."

Most attorneys are not counselors. Before you consult an attorney, you will want to sit down with a counselor or trusted friends and decide what kind of a family you want for your baby and if you want an open adoption.

In a private adoption, the adopting couple pay for all of the medical expenses incurred during the pregnancy, including the monthly checkups by a gynecologist and the hospital delivery. The couple also pays the attorney's fees.

Because the adopting couple is involved from the start, they begin building up a storehouse of love for that unknown infant. One of the most heart-wrenching things a birth mother can do is decide to take back the child at the last minute. The adopting couple will feel like they just lost their child and go through an intense grieving process. After all, they had prepared their hearts to receive the child, investing a great deal of time, money, and emotions in the process.

Adoption is not to be entered into lightly, without thought. The birth mother should attempt to make a careful decision before the birth. In that way she will protect herself as well as the adopting couple from needless pain.

If a birth mother does decide to reverse her decision and keep the child, she must be prepared to face a whole new batch of decisions and complications as a single mother.

Agency Adoption

Many county, state, and private agencies exist to help place children in homes. Birth mothers are often afraid to go through agencies because they believe their child will be lost in a paperwork shuffle and they will lose control over the type of family the child will be raised in. Some agencies are not reputable. Some agencies place the infant in a foster home for months before actual placement in a family. However, some are excellent and should be considered. Do not be afraid to have other people check out the agency before you decide. Most pregnant girls are in far too emotional a state to think very clearly. Get others to help you locate a reputable agency.

Open Adoption

Many young birth mothers choose open adoption because it gives them so much control over placement and visiting rights. Some open adoptions consist of the birth mother meeting the adopting parents and then arranging for a letter and a picture of the child to be sent on an annual basis. This helps the birth mother feel like her child is well off and lessens the wondering about her child in later years. Other open adoptions give the birth mother extensive visiting rights to the child. Most open adoptions work out very well.

One caution needs to be kept in mind here. Once the child is released for adoption, that child is no longer yours. It belongs to another family—legally, socially, physically, and emotionally.

Now that you've gone over what types of adoption are available, you can see that releasing a child for adoption is not letting go of your responsibility. It's the beginning of taking responsibility for your life and the life of your child.

Fruit of My Body, Sin of My Soul

Shall I offer my firstborn for my transgression, the fruit of my body for the sin of my soul?

Micah 6:7b

"Nurse."

"What is it?"

"I want to see my baby, please."

(Long pause)

"I'm sorry. It's just not convenient at this time."

A little while later I tried again. Pressing the buzzer beside the hospital bed I lay there, listening to a different nurse answer over the intercom.

"I want to see my baby, please."

"I'm sorry but the doctor thinks it best that you don't see her."

"Well, I think I want to see her," I said, adding a note of force to my shaky voice as I began to grow angry.

"We can't bring her to the room right now. I'll check with the doctor and see what he says."

My face reddened as I left my bed determined to have a look at the infant I had brought into the world less than twenty-four hours ago. I threw my blanket on the floor, walked to the closet, and ripped out the new bathrobe my mother had bought for my hospital stay. Pulling it over that skimpy hospital gown so my backside wouldn't show, I began my long march down the corridor, past the nurses' station and around the corner to stand in front of the nursery window. Which one was she? Where was she? They all looked so much alike. I had only held my baby for a moment in the delivery room before the nurse took her away, and I knew I could not pick her out. None of the infants had names labeling their cribs. Little heads and swaddled bodies rippled behind pools of water forming in my eyes. Mouths sucking empty air. I heard feeble cries. Rows of infants with mothers. Vacant cribs where loving hands had claimed their bundles and settled into homes and families. The tears began to roll down my cheeks.

A nurse tending the infants turned around and stared at me, bewildered. Without saying a word to me, she disappeared behind a partition.

For three days I lay in the hospital and cried. On the third day, my mother came into the room and said, "The adopting couple are here for the child, so let's stay for a moment and pack your things before we leave."

As we drove home, I was hoping it was all over now and that my body would resume its normal shape and life would go on as planned. But somehow, I sensed I would never be the same.

It was November of my senior year in high school when I began feeling different. Pretty soon, I realized that my periods had ceased. My stomach felt a little harder, while my breasts and cheeks grew puffier.

I did what most girls do when they think they are pregnant. I called my best friend. She gave me the phone number of a free pregnancy testing clinic located in a small office building in a nearby city. Ditching school, I rode the bus the next day and found the address. I felt really sleazy walking into the slummy part of town, as if I were a teenage hooker.

At the clinic, a woman handed me a vial and a piece of paper and said, "Urinate into the cup and write on the paper, and I'll be out in a moment to collect them."

Brief and to the point, I thought as I walked into the tiny restroom. I knew deep inside that I was pregnant, but I desperately hoped it wasn't true, that the test would be negative. So I peed in the cup and wrote out the information, and the woman eventually came out to collect them. She said they would call me the next day with the result.

They called. My test was negative. I was not pregnant—according to the test.

But I knew the test was wrong. Wanting to believe the results, however, I entered into a dreamlike state of denial and waited.

Denial is the first symptom of any problem too large to handle. Unplanned pregnancy, for most teenagers, is too hard to cope with initially. So denial kicks in and we say, "This problem doesn't exist." Fantasy thoughts breeze through one's mind and blow away all realistic thinking: it can't happen to me . . . virgins can't get pregnant . . . no one gets pregnant the first time . . . my periods weren't regular enough to get pregnant. However, reality is that anyone can get pregnant the first time, no matter how young you are.

In my denial stage I became very quiet and spent lots of time walking on the beach listening to the hypnotic pounding of the surf and thinking about absolutely nothing. I began to think of the ocean as a giant womb full of life, always pregnant. I began to feel like I would always be pregnant and never give birth. I carried all sorts of strange ideas inside my head and they seemed to build into even larger and stranger ideas before I told anyone my secret.

For at least four months I kept my secret. One day, my mother suggested that I go to the doctor because I seemed to be gaining a little weight. I agreed.

There in the office the doctor felt my abdomen very seriously. "Well," he said with a great fatherly smile, "it looks like you've got something to be proud of. I would say that you are going to have a baby."

I didn't want to hear that. I wasn't proud of being pregnant and not in the least happy. All I could think of was how to tell my mother when I got home. The doctor offered to tell her for me, but I said I could do it myself. He gave me the name of an obstetrician-gynecologist (ob/gyn) and told me to make an appointment for monthly checkups during the pregnancy. I had no idea what an ob-gyn was and I didn't ask. I found out later that they are doctors that specialize in the female reproductive system and deliver babies.

I don't remember driving home. When I walked in the front door I saw my mother sitting on the couch. She looked up and asked what the doctor had to say. A long moment of silence hung thickly in the air while I struggled for the right words to say. Finally, I blurted out, "Mom, I'm pregnant," and burst into tears.

My mother sat stunned for a moment. Then she got up and gave me one of her rare hugs, one of those arm-around-the-shoulders-and-side-squeeze hugs. Not a big happy hug like she was pleased with the occasion. Just a sympathy hug while I sobbed. After a while, she suggested I go to bed. I slept for hours, relieved that I no longer had to carry my secret alone.

Later that evening, my dad came in and woke me up. Sitting on the edge of the bed, he put his arms around me and let me cry some more.

The dreamlike state of denial lifted, and I began to consider my options. The decision-making process was more difficult than I'd imagined. I ruled out abortion because the doctor informed me that abortions were unsafe after the first trimester (the first three months of pregnancy). Besides, I sensed that I had a person growing inside of me, and that made me responsible for someone else's life. I decided to carry the baby to term. Then I realized that I had better start taking care of my body so the baby wouldn't get sick. I quit smoking those occasional cigarettes that now made me nauseous. I stopped drinking alcohol and stayed away from anyone smoking pot. For the first time in my life, I was considering the welfare of another person over my own.

I still couldn't decide whether to keep the baby when she was born or release her for adoption. And I still hadn't told my boyfriend about the situation. We had only had sex once. It happened one night when I got into a huge fight with my mother. I ran out of the house, slamming the door behind me. I walked to a nearby phone booth and called my boyfriend Paul to come pick me up. And I spent the night at his house.

I had known Paul for about six months and nick-named him "the intellectual party animal." I liked him more and more as the days passed. But the morning after I spent the night with him our relationship changed. I didn't like him anymore.

I found out later that many couples split up after they have sex. They can't seem to stand each other afterward, maybe because they weren't ready for the commitment sex implies. Couples at my high school that I thought were so in love and headed for marriage broke up after they had gone "all the way." Paul and I were no different.

As soon as I found out I was pregnant, I started hating him. He kept calling me, wondering why I wouldn't go out with him anymore.

One day, I went over to his apartment to tell him.

He put away his college calculus text, looked up, and said, "Are you sure?"

Then he said, "What about an abortion? I'll pay for it all."

After I said it was too late for an abortion, he thought for a moment and said, "OK, why don't you move in with me until you have the baby?"

When I questioned him as to what we would do after the baby was born he said we could raise it together.

Right.

I told him I didn't want to see him again, that I was going to put the baby up for adoption.

"Look," he said, getting really mad, "I want that

baby. It's just as much mine as it is yours. If you don't move in with me I'll take the baby and raise it."

I couldn't believe what I had just heard. Paul, want the baby? I imagined him changing diapers and smoking a joint, then putting the child to bed and inviting a few of his buddies over for a party. I shook my head.

What a fight we had that night. And I realized beyond all doubt that neither of us were ready for parenthood.

Seven months pregnant, I went forward to receive my high school diploma. No one ever acknowledged my pregnancy because I wore very loose T-shirts that hung over my jeans, and I kept my presence at school to a minimum—to such a minimum that sometimes I felt as though I didn't even exist. It was an eerie feeling.

After a couple of talks with my mother I decided I was not cut out to be a single mother. I couldn't support myself, much less a child. I had other plans for life than changing diapers, nursing a sick kid who cried all night, and struggling to pay bills and baby-sitters. So, during the last three months of my pregnancy, I was busy with attorneys trying to set up a private adoption.

One evening, my father came home and said he had made an appointment for me to talk to an attorney who specialized in arranging adoptions.

The moment I walked into this attorney's office I hated him. He looked like a big, fat baby seller to me. I imagined my dad plopping open the yellow pages and looking under "Baby Seller" to find this guy. From the looks of his office, he made a great living trafficking in babies. And from the looks of his glance—cold and businesslike—he seemed to care little for the birth mother. I could see dollar signs ringing up in his eyes when I walked into the room.

To make things worse, he was one of those men who hunts animals so he can stuff their heads and display them as trophies of his masculinity. The heads of a deer, gazelle, moose, and even a tiger stared down at me from their mounts on the redwood paneled walls of the office.

I dubbed the lawyer the "Big Game Hunter." There he sat, leaning back in his dark, leather chair, rolls of fat oozing over his belt. *He's got to be a fake*, I thought. *How could he possibly get his fat butt into the jungle to shoot all of these?*

"What can I do for you?" he asked.

What do you think we're here for? I sneered silently, *so you can hunt me down and hang my head on your wall?* I let my parents answer his question, explaining the situation as if the attorney were blind to my protruding belly.

My attention drifted as I gazed around the office. The more my eyes lingered on the gazelle, the moose, the tiger, the more I sensed this lawyer's disregard for the individual and the dignity of life. He didn't seem to care that I was ready to entrust my flesh and blood to another human being. He didn't care that I was scared, that I faced a difficult decision. In fact, he didn't care about me at all. All he cared about was the money.

He turned his fleshy cheeks toward me and started firing questions, barely looking at me as he wrote my answers down. Apparently, the adoption was in progress.

"Wait a minute!" I interrupted rudely. "I don't want to deal with you. I don't like you, and as far as I'm concerned, you're not getting anything from me, because I can see you don't give a damn about anyone." Shaking, I rose from my seat and turned to my parents. "Come on. We're getting out of here." I slammed out of that office without apology.

It's one thing to decide to release a child for adoption. It's more difficult to actually follow through with the plan.

The next attorney was a woman handling her first adoption case—mine. As is often the case, the attorney knew of a couple who wanted to adopt but promised to obtain other information about adopting couples so I would have a choice. I liked her. If she highly recommended the adopting couple, I felt like I could trust her judgment. We met a couple of times and she asked me all sorts of embarrassing questions like did I ever take drugs and what kind, was I sure about the baby's father (was he really Asian or was he black . . . or was he an alien from outer space), and what kind of family did I want for my baby. That part of the process was very uncomfortable. But I also had the opportunity to ask all sorts of questions about the adoption process and the couple who were going to adopt my child. As the days went by, I began to realize that the baby would cease to be mine and belong—emotionally, physically, and legally—to the adopting couple.

The hospital experience seemed like one quick rush of pain, blurred nurses, a metal bed, X-rays. All systems were go. It was delivery time.

I looked up into the ceiling mirror positioned so that I could watch the birth. The doctor kept up a steady stream of chatter, directing me when to push and when to relax, announcing what was going on as if he were a sports announcer calling the latest score.

Finally, a tiny head peeked through, and a moment later, the rest of the body slid into the doctor's hands. He cut the umbilical cord and said, "Congratulations. It's a girl." The pain was over. Within a couple of minutes, the nurse placed the child in my arms, and we created our one brief memory of life together.

Two days later the adoptive couple came to the hospital and the child vanished out of my life and entered into theirs.

Like many girls who release their children for adoption, I went through a period of feeling numb and empty. Little did I know that many women, after giving birth, undergo a time of the blues, called postpartum depression. But those who have abortions or release children for adoption compound their sadness, going through the stages of grief that accompany great loss or the death of someone you love.

As a defense against the grieving process I did what most do: I refused to think about the situation or what I had just been through. But I lived with a nagging sense of guilt and sadness that got worse around the time of my baby's birthday, a feeling called the "Anniversary Syndrome." Eventually, I knew I had to talk about it with someone. The guilt was driving me crazy.

By then, I had heard enough about Jesus Christ to believe that he was the God who loved me, created me, and established a plan for my life before I was even born. The guilt was beginning to lift, but all sorts of other feelings surfaced as a result. I had shoved the whole experience so deep into the basement of my mind that it seemed like a dream long past. Questions assaulted my mind. Who really adopted her? Was it just a dream or did it really happen? Where was she? What did she look like? How could anybody love me after what I had done?

I realized that I needed help to sort through all these thoughts and emotions. So I went to visit a friend of mine from church. It was the first time I had shared the whole story with someone. She listened for hours. As I talked, the tears flowed, the craziness of my thoughts poured out, and the guilt subsided. My story over, she offered to pray for me that God would heal the pain and release me from the guilt I still felt.

"Holy Spirit, you are the comforter. Come and bring your comfort and healing to this mother's heart," she prayed simply.

And God responded. His presence surrounded me, wrapping me in loving warmth like a blanket. I felt so peaceful that I fell into a dream for a brief moment. I saw myself in the delivery room giving birth, a final

Fruit of My Body, Sin of My Soul

push sliding the infant into the doctor's hands. Looking at the doctor as he pulled the mask down from his nose and mouth, I recognized the face of Jesus.

"I have her," he said. "I took her."

"You what?" I cried in disbelief.

"I have her," he gently replied.

I began to weep with relief, each tear releasing more of the anger, guilt, and sadness that I had carried for so long. I realized that Jesus was with me the whole miserable time, even before I knew who he was.

And then I knew what he meant when he said, "I have her." His eye watches over her life as well as mine, guiding us both, caring for us both, loving us both, and raising us both as only a perfect father can. And then Christ's love filled the void that my baby had left behind.

The Note on the Mirror

Mom,

I can't face you. I don't know what to do so I'm leaving
this note on your bathroom mirror. I'm pregnant. If you want
to call and talk to me I'm at my girlfriend Joni's.

Telling your parents that you're pregnant is one of the most difficult
things you'll ever do. Once your parents know, everyone seems to get
involved—brothers and sisters, grandparents, your boyfriend, his brothers
and sisters, and his parents and grandparents. Where does it all end?
Everyone wants either to ignore the situation or exert their control. Friends
don't know what to say and avoid you. Your boyfriend says cruel things
and shrugs off responsibilities he is not prepared to take. Once the news is
out in the open, you're off on an emotional roller coaster that doesn't
seem to want to stop.

Melia's story reveals just how much others are affected when they hear
someone they love say, "I'm pregnant."

When Melia first discovered she was pregnant, she
denied it. *This isn't happening,* she thought. *It isn't
true. Something is going to happen that will make all of
this go away. It will all be over and I won't have to deal
with it. My parents will never have to know.*

But her parents did have to find out some day. After
all, Melia was over four months pregnant, and her
weight gain was growing noticeable. Usually Melia
would just brush her problems onto someone else or
someone would bail her out. But this time *she* had to
handle the situation.

She thought about having an abortion but it was too
late, too risky, and too costly. She ignored the symptoms

of pregnancy so long that an X-ray could reveal the form of a tiny infant sucking its thumb within her womb.

Melia was six months pregnant when she told her mother. One morning she left a note that said, "I can't face you. I don't know what to do so I'm leaving this note on your bathroom mirror. I'm pregnant. If you want to call me and talk to me I'm over at my girlfriend Joni's." Then she went to Joni's and sat there for hours, wondering when her mother would find the note and call. It was about three in the afternoon when she finally called and asked Melia to come home.

When Melia came home, she saw that her mother was crying. Her mother didn't seem to know what to do or say. Neither of them spoke. Then her mother said, "So, how did this happen?"

"What did she expect me to say? Explain the facts of life as I knew it?" She started to cry.

They had barely begun talking when Melia's stepdad walked in. Her mother looked at him and said, "We have a problem."

"What is it?" he asked. He was the one Melia really didn't want to tell. As soon as he walked in the door, she started bawling some more.

Melia's mother told her stepdad that Melia was pregnant.

It didn't faze Melia's stepdad a bit. He said he knew. How could he not know? Melia was six months pregnant and noticeably fat, even though she wore sweats to cover up. But he and her mother had both silently decided to ignore all the telltale signs of pregnancy and pretend it would just go away.

Finally faced with the reality of the situation, her parents asked Melia why she didn't use birth control. Melia didn't know. She said to me, "You see those sex education movies in elementary school, but you don't realize anyone is really having sex. And you especially don't think you ever are going to have sex. But you do it.

And afterward, you panic, wondering if you're pregnant and counting the days until your period."

Like Melia, many girls operate on the "do it first and worry later" motto of the fool. They know when they are heading into a sexual encounter, but they push it out of their mind instead of choosing how they will respond. If they had thought about the consequences of sex ahead of time, they might have stayed out of the situation in the first place, saving themselves a lot of grief.

The next grief Melia faced was telling her boyfriend. She had met Eric in junior high and began going out with him a few years later. When they were alone together, he treated her well, but once he was in the company of his friends, he acted as if he didn't know her. They broke up many times, only to get back together again. Melia kept hoping Eric would change and really fall in love with her.

One night Melia saw Eric at a party. They decided to leave together. Melia said, "Why we were even together that night I'll never know. We were coming home from the party and it just happened. I don't remember thinking in advance, 'I think I'll have sex tonight.' That's why you don't think about birth control ... because you don't plan on it happening. We had been drinking quite a bit at the party and it just happened."

Funny how a lot of things "just happen" when you're drinking. Alcohol tends to lower inhibitions. It sweeps into the brain like a fog, erasing rational thoughts, scrambling all your emotions, and toying with your physiological responses. Remember your first drink? Those few beers made you dizzy, happy; it made everything seem funny or profound. You probably believed that the guy you met at the party fell madly in love with you. Maybe you gave in and had sex. And the next day, you started worrying about being pregnant.

For Melia, "it just happened" meant they were pretty

buzzed. They drank enough to let themselves get out of control.

After she discovered she was pregnant, Melia called Eric. "Can't be mine," he said. "I'm sterile. Take me to court and order a blood test if you want to. But it's not mine."

She told him that she wasn't making it up and it wasn't a ploy to get back together with him as a boyfriend. She just didn't want to be the only one going through the pregnancy. She wanted Eric to know so that he could take on his share of the suffering.

But he continued to refuse to have anything to do with the pregnancy. Finally, Melia hung up on him, crushed by his callousness. She felt like packing her bags and hitchhiking out of town. But what would she do then? Feeling trapped and very much alone, she decided to stay, live at home, and wait for the baby to be born.

After a while, Melia was on the blackball list at school. Everyone knew she was pregnant. The vice principal called her into her office and said she knew about Melia's pregnancy. She told Melia about the district's teen mother program, a special school program that would allow Melia to finish her education without having to deal with the comments and stares of other students.

Melia decided to try out the program. But the realities of teenage motherhood hit her the first day she walked into class. The principal hadn't told her that all the girls in that class were going to keep their babies. Melia was not at all sure she was going to keep her baby, but there she was in a program full of pregnant girls learning how to feed, diaper, and care for their babies. She walked out and never went back.

Unknown to Melia, her mother realized that she wasn't going to face reality and get prepared for motherhood. She assumed that Melia was headed in the direction of adoption and began talking to friends about adoption procedures. Then she confronted Melia with the information. She asked Melia a list of questions. Did she want to be a single parent? How was she going to support the child? What did she know about caring for sick infants? It dawned on Melia that she didn't have a clue about how to be a parent. Nor did she want to raise the child.

It was a rude awakening for Melia. Because she hadn't made a decision during the past few months of her pregnancy, her options were narrowing. Her mother called her real father and told him Melia was pregnant. He offered financial assistance to her if she chose to raise the child. Her grandparents also offered to help and presented her with an opportunity to keep the baby. Now Melia was forced to make a final decision: Keep the child, or release her for adoption? Either way, the decision was hers.

Melia decided to go for the adoption process. Her mother handled everything, finding an attorney through a friend of hers who had adopted a child.

Melia described her pregnancy to me. "The more I felt her move inside of me, the more difficult it got for me to let her go," she said. "It's a great feeling, being pregnant, and every time you feel the baby move you want the baby to stay there and not come out. I didn't know what was going to happen to us once she was born. I didn't know where she was going to be. I kept fighting all of the questions of the unknown. I wanted to stay at home and be pregnant forever, just to keep the feeling of life inside of me. But I was scared, because I knew that after she was born I would probably never see her again."

Melia went into labor in the middle of the night. By 7:30 A.M., her daughter was born. It was time for Melia to release her baby into the hands of the adopting

The Note on the Mirror

couple who would nurture, love, and raise the child as if she were their own.

Like most birth mothers, Melia had her last-minute doubts. But she followed through on her decision despite her longing to keep her daughter after she was born.

Melia's parents and family also grieved the loss of their granddaughter, their niece. Sympathizing with the pain Melia was feeling, her sister retaliated against Eric. As soon as the baby was born, she called Eric's house. His mother answered the phone and said Eric wasn't there. Melia's sister announced, "I was calling to tell him that his daughter was just born. It's too bad you'll never be able to see your granddaughter." Eric's mother had no idea that her son was a father. She began yelling out questions to her unknown caller, but Melia's sister hung up without answering. Eric was in for a surprise confrontation when he came home that day. And his parents began dealing with all the thoughts and feelings of having a grandchild they would never know.

While Melia was in the hospital, Eric called and said he was coming to see her and that he felt bad about the whole thing. Before he hung up, he reminded her that she couldn't keep the baby. He didn't want Melia to trap him into a responsibility that he wasn't ready to undertake. Eric never showed up at the hospital, and Melia was bitterly hurt.

The only other contact Melia had with Eric came a year later when it was time to sign the final adoption papers. He told her he couldn't make it to the county social worker's office to sign the papers. He had other plans. Melia went alone.

The social worker acted insensitively. When Melia started crying in his office, giving him a hard time about signing the papers, he got angry. He stomped out of the room to get her a tissue. While he was gone, Melia snuck a look through her file to see if there was a birth certificate with her baby's name on it and the names of the adopting parents. She saw their address and wrote it down, but she later lost it. She was curious about what was written about her, but there wasn't time to read it all before the social worker came back.

Melia could have worked out an adoption agreement before she gave birth that would have allowed her to see her child. At the very least, she could have requested an annual update about her daughter by receiving a letter and a picture. She even declined the opportunity to meet the adopting couple because of her own fears. She might have been better off if she had met her fears head on and taken more responsibility in the decision-making process. She would have had less to wonder about later on.

Shortly after Melia signed the papers, Eric took his turn. Melia followed him in her car to make sure he followed through. He went into the office alone while Melia waited in the parking lot. When he came out he was crying. He kicked the car a few times, trying to vent all of the feelings that he had ignored for over a year. Melia realized for the first time how much Eric was affected as he realized that it was his child too. They had never talked about giving the baby up for adoption. All Eric said was that she couldn't keep it. Now, there he was in the parking lot saying, "I can't believe it. All I had to do was sign my name on a piece of paper."

Melia got angry. Describing the situation to me, she said, "Eric didn't have to go through half of what I went through." But Eric had his own feelings to deal with as he realized that he had lost a part of himself in that baby. The birth mother is not the only one affected by a baby's birth and adoption. The birth father is affected more than anyone realizes.

A Letter and a Picture

It's never too late to release a child for adoption. Coping with household bills and meeting the constant demands of a needy infant alone are not easy tasks by any means. Dreams of finding a husband who will rise to the occasion of fatherhood dwindle as the single mother faces the burdens of daily life. As fear begins to swallow all hope for the future, some young women feel the stress of motherhood frazzling their nerves to the breaking point. They can't go it alone any longer.

Linda was one of these mothers. At first Linda didn't think there was much to know about being a mother. After all, babies only drank milk and messed their diapers. You hire a baby-sitter or drop the kid off at Mom's every time you want to go out on a date. Really, life isn't interrupted too much.

When Linda's son David was only a few months old, people began to point out to Linda the little things that mothers do to care for their infants. One friend pointed out to her that she needed to sterilize David's bottles—they stank. Linda started to notice other things that mothers should do, things she wasn't doing. She began to feel like an unfit mother when, in truth, she was an unlearned mother.

All this time Linda's mother and stepfather never pointed out the problems with Linda's ability as a mom, but they did offer suggestions and discreet hints. For example, they kept offering to take David if Linda planned to go out that night. When David stayed with other baby-sitters they discreetly asked Linda who was baby-sitting. Their questions about her baby-sitters led Linda to realize that she didn't care who stayed with David. She knew nothing about screening baby-sitters and laying out guidelines for them. So David stayed with grandmother quite often while Linda went to work or went out at night in search of Mr. Right.

Occasionally, she would invite someone over for dinner, imagining a cozy, candlelit dinner for two. But there was David, acting like the infant he was, demanding attention, crying for dinner, messing his pants, and refusing to fall asleep later on. David spoiled many evenings, and Linda's annoyance grew. Finally, however, the dinner dates paid off. Linda's dreams of finding a husband and a father for David were starting to come true. She got engaged to a man named Jim. Everything was going to be all right now.

Perhaps Jim felt more pity for Linda than love. He began to dread the responsibilities of being a father, and he sought counsel from his former Christian youth group leaders. They assured him that he didn't have to feel forced into fatherhood. It was the out he was looking for. He broke off the engagement. Linda's hopes of being a "good Christian wife and mother" shattered, and despair filled her heart.

Linda described this time in her life to me. "I figured I didn't know how to be a mother and David would never have a father," she said. "My patience grew thinner and thinner when he cried in the middle of the night and I didn't want to get out of bed. I would say, 'Why do you want to get up, David? Go back to sleep' and leave him there until I felt like getting up. Sometimes he would lie there for a couple of hours, hungry and wet, until I got up."

Linda's failures as a mother began to haunt her, tormenting her with guilt. Her thinking grew so warped that she started thinking her son would be better off dead.

One day, Linda turned on the tap, intending to draw a bath for her ten-month-old son. The tormenting thoughts bombarded her once more: *David would be better off dead . . . You're an unfit mother . . . Look at*

A Letter and a Picture

what you do to him ... You don't even know how to take care of him ... She left the water running in the tub, put David in with a few toys, and quietly left the house.

A couple of hours later, she walked back into her apartment expecting to find her son drowned. Instead, David stood upright, a big grin on his face, one hand holding onto the faucet. "Hi mama. Wawa," he said as he splashed away with his free hand. Water ran over the sides of the tub, spilling onto the bathroom floor.

When Linda saw her son, still alive and well, she knew she wasn't ready to be a mother. She took him out of the tub and wrapped a towel around him, holding him and rocking him, crying as she said over and over, "I'm sorry ... I'm sorry." At that moment, she began seriously considering giving David up for adoption.

If Linda hadn't made that decision, someone would have made it for her. Had David drowned, Linda probably would have gone to jail. Murdering a child carries a long prison sentence. Abandoning an infant by leaving it in a trash can or on somebody's doorstep is also illegal. Mothers like Linda who can't cope had better ask for help before they reach the breaking point.

This was the last in a series of breaking points for Linda. Each time God had miraculously intervened to spare David's life. First God foiled Linda's attempt to get an abortion. Then he prevented her suicide when she was pregnant with David. And now this. No ten-month-old child has the stamina to hold onto a faucet for long. One slip and the infant would have had a great deal of difficulty getting back on his feet. Children drown in as little as six inches of water. God's hand was definitely on David's life. But he also protected Linda every step of the way.

Linda was sixteen years old the summer she decided to run away from her home in Washington state to follow her boyfriend, Larry, whose family had just moved to

Texas. Until that time, Linda's reputation as a "good Christian girl" was engraved on the hearts and minds of all her teachers and friends at the Christian school she and Larry attended. No one could imagine Linda running off.

But after Larry left, something in Linda broke. She loved him and couldn't deal with living apart from him. So she ran away to be with him, and it was a couple of weeks before her parents tracked her down and sent the police for her. The police dropped her off at a home for runaways, a prison complete with bars on the windows. She stayed there a few days, until her parents decided Linda could stay with Larry and his parents and called to have her released.

As Linda got ready to leave the home, one of the women said, "Don't get pregnant." Larry's mother was there, and she replied, "These are good kids. We don't have to worry about them."

But good kids have sexual desires too. Within a week, Linda and Larry were sleeping together. They knew that what they were doing was wrong, but since they planned on getting married they didn't feel guilty, even when they went to church or their youth group. Linda lived in her own little world, planning to marry Larry in a nearby state where sixteen was the legal marriage age.

Pretty soon, Linda and Larry were having sex on a regular basis. Linda began to have a nagging feeling that she was pregnant. Not only that, but something was happening to Larry, too. Mr. Nice Guy was turning into a jealous maniac.

One night, Larry stayed home from the church youth meeting and Linda went alone. Afterward, the youth group went over to someone's house to play video games and eat popcorn. When the evening was over, one of the guys drove Linda home. Larry came flying out of the house hysterical because another guy was driving Linda home. He demanded to know what they were doing and where they had been. Having grown up with a violent father, Linda knew immediately what was happening. The last thing Linda wanted to endure was the kind of abuse she'd grown up with. She resolved to leave Larry.

Given the situation, Linda acted wisely. Living with an abusive boyfriend is dangerous. One of the first clues that a man may become physically violent is jealousy and possessiveness. Larry was headed into a pattern of violence: verbal abuse, flying into a rage, and wanting Linda all to himself. Pretty soon, he would have forbidden Linda to go anywhere without him. If she did go somewhere without him, every time she came home Larry would have drilled her with jealous questions. Perhaps he even would have hit her as he created false accusations born out of his own crazy imagination. Eventually, the violence would worsen until Linda would have been trapped . . . maybe even dead. If your boyfriend is the jealous type, watch out! True love is not jealous or possessive. True love is shown by a kiss on the cheek, not a slap across the face.

The next morning, Linda packed her bags and called her mother from a neighbor's house. Her mother contacted the only people she could think of to help: the Salvation Army, a church with branches located everywhere. A man with the Salvation Army had helped Linda's mom out when she fled from her abusive husband, so she thought to call the Texas branch. Sure enough, the Salvation Army sent a man dressed in his uniform to the neighbor's house to pick up Linda. He drove her to a hotel, gave her a plane ticket, and instructed her to take the airport shuttle the next morning for her flight home.

Once home, Linda told her mom she thought she was pregnant. Sure enough, a home pregnancy test confirmed it, and a series of decisions had to be made. After telling her stepfather the news, she left home, moving into a friend's apartment. A few days later, she called a former boyfriend and asked him to help her arrange for an abortion. She was about two months pregnant at the time. He agreed to help and said he would be over in the morning to drive her to the abortion clinic.

But God had other plans for Linda. Her friend stopped off at a woman's house on his way to pick up Linda. She said to him, "If you take her to get an abortion, you are going to be responsible for that child's life. That child's blood is going to be on your head." The woman was a Christian who knew both Linda and her friend. After that conversation, he couldn't go through with his plans. He never showed up at Linda's apartment. David's life was spared . . . miracle number one.

Miracle number two came hard on the heels of the first miracle. Later that afternoon, Linda tried to commit suicide. Deeply depressed, she felt as though she had ruined everyone's life. Her stepfather had acted as though she were the ungrateful child who messed up the family's reputation. She couldn't get a ride to the abortion clinic. She didn't know where to turn or what else to do.

Drunk when she attempted suicide, Linda swallowed a handful of pills. She thought she would die quickly. Instead, the combination caused her to vomit immediately, expelling the drugs from her system. She kept vomiting. Reaching for the phone, she called her parents, who sent the paramedics to the apartment. She was sick for two weeks after failing the suicide attempt. A friend of her parents took her in and nursed her back to health.

Some people attempt suicide as a cry for help without thinking of what will happen if they fail. Others attempt suicide, not to cry for help, but because they really want to die. They are so depressed that they see nothing but

A Letter and a Picture

darkness surrounding them. To them, dying is just stepping from one darkness into another. They reach the point where they cannot think about anything rationally: People they love, hopes for a better tomorrow, thoughts of ending up in heaven or hell don't exist. They just feel overwhelming pain and their struggle for the moment.

In Linda's case, she was crying out for help. And God listened, reaching out his hand to protect her. Not only did he save her from death; he also kept the combination of pills and alcohol from chemically scrambling her brain, for the combination she took was enough to send her into a coma and cause permanent brain damage.

As Linda came out of the fog of depression and sickness caused by the suicide attempt, she felt an urging deep within to release her child for adoption. She decided that if he were a boy she would name him David, beloved gift of God, and that he would go to another family. She began seeking more knowledge about this God she sensed working in her life and started reading the Bible. She read the story of Hannah in the book of Samuel and saw how God had used the adoption of Samuel to accomplish great things. However, as the time drew closer for David's birth, Linda changed her mind. She decided to keep her baby.

Linda's parents threw her a baby shower and rallied to her support. Now that she was outfitted for raising a baby, she thought she was set. There wasn't anything to raising a baby. After all, the instructions to everything were on the packages.

Motherhood came as a complete shock. Sterilize bottles? Crying at 3:00 A.M.? Why not feed him peanut butter at two months old? How about a steak? Linda found that she didn't know the first thing about being a mother. Then the day came when Linda drew the bath. She had reached the breaking point.

Linda dried David off and dressed him. Then she

called her former church youth leaders, Ron and Patty, and told them she was ready to give David up. Patty could tell from her voice that the situation was serious and suggested that it be done right away. She told Linda she would come over to the sitter's the next morning and pick David up before Linda could change her mind, as she'd done so many times before.

The next morning Linda kissed David, putting his hat on as slowly as she could. Her boyfriend John came to take him to the sitter's. That was the last time she saw David.

Linda had been told by Ron and Patty that he would be placed with a loving family during the adoption process. Later on, she discovered that the loving family was her own parents. David had a final week with his grandparents until the adoption papers were signed. As she signed the papers, Linda realized that she was relinquishing David for the rest of his life. She cried the whole time she was in the attorney's office.

"It was very hard," Linda said. "When I finally decided to let him go, I wrote notes to give to the adopting couple about what kind of food David liked, things he liked to play with, books he liked me to read to him. I sent everything I had of his with him because I wanted him to have some familiar toys. I was concerned he would wake up and not know where he was, and it was a way of making me feel better."

Linda made a verbal agreement with the adopting couple that they would send a letter and a picture once a year so she would know how David was doing. The following year, she received a letter and a picture. She was comforted by them and felt like she had done the right thing.

But the next year, nothing came. No letter, no picture. Linda found out from Ron and Patty that the adopting couple were afraid Linda would recognize David from the photos and one day want to come and get him. In addition, the couple thought that Linda, having further contact with David, would threaten his adjustment. Linda was crushed.

Linda turned to God during this time for her strength, and he built up her faith. She began to realize that she had given her son not just to Steve and Diana, the adopting couple, but to the Lord, just as Hannah had in the Bible. "God showed me that every one of us is adopted," Linda said. "As soon as we accept Jesus as our Savior, we are adopted into the family of God. God becomes our true Father.

"When I gave David to the Lord, he took David and handed him to Steve and Diana, knowing that they could love David for him. And when I cried out to the Lord, 'Love David for me,' he replied, 'I am. This is the way I am loving him . . . through Steve and Diana.' When I saw that, I didn't think of David as being my son anymore. He was just a gift I received from God and gave back to God. And God shared him with someone else. Then I wasn't so hurt that Steve and Diana had stopped sharing David with me."

Adoption: Step-by-Step

1. FIND OUT IF YOU ARE PREGNANT.

Drugstores carry a variety of home pregnancy tests that can be purchased by anyone, regardless of age. Generally the tests are reliable, but any test results should be confirmed by a doctor. If you are too embarrassed to buy a home pregnancy test kit, arrange to have a confidential test done at a crisis pregnancy clinic. Phone numbers for local clinics are found in the yellow pages of your phone book. The telephone operator can also locate a pregnancy clinic in a town near you.

If you are stuck, call one of the numbers listed below. There is no charge for a phone call that starts with an 800 number, and it won't show up on your parents' phone bill. Ask them where you can have a pregnancy test done in your area.

Lifeline	1 (800) 238-4269
National Pregnancy Hotline	1 (800) 344-7211
Birthright (U.S. & Canada)	1 (800) 328-LOVE
The Pearson Foundation (Catholic)	1 (800) 633-2252 ext. 700

2. CALL A PREGNANCY COUNSELOR.

You don't have to struggle alone. By calling one of the above hotline numbers you can get in touch with people who are equipped to listen to you without pressuring you into a decision. The person who answers the phone will refer you to people who live close by. Contact that person. It will most likely be a woman who will offer a great deal of emotional support and help you in many ways. Most crisis pregnancy counselors can provide the following assistance:

- pregnancy counseling
- financial assistance for medical problems
- community assistance for financial needs
- residential care (if your parents ask you to leave home while you are pregnant or you can't stand to stay home, they will find a place for you to stay)
- information on where to go for pregnancy tests and further counseling
- adoption services
- infant foster care (temporary care for your baby while you decide whether to parent or while you make final adoption plans)

Don't be afraid to call. The counselors know how difficult this situation is for you and will help you talk about it. Sometimes it's easier to talk to a total stranger.

3. LIST THE PEOPLE YOU FEEL YOU CAN TRUST TO HELP.

You don't have to worry about being pregnant and alone. List some people you can talk to: friends, your mother, someone else's mother, a teacher, a youth group leader. This may be the time to let your secret out and allow others to stand by you. You may be surprised at what you discover. Those who you think will understand may not know how to deal with the news or know how to help you. People who you think will absolutely freak out may be the ones who handle it best. Don't write your parents off out of fear of how they will respond. They are going to find out sooner or later. It may as well be from the beginning.

4. EXPLORE YOUR OPTIONS.

You must be doing that or you wouldn't be reading this book. That's great. Ultimately, the decision of what you are going to do is yours alone. People may help you, but no one can make up your mind about going the adoption route or deciding to parent.

5. ARRANGE FOR ONGOING DOCTOR'S APPOINTMENTS.

This will ensure that you and the baby remain healthy during your pregnancy. Your counselor from the crisis pregnancy center can help you with this.

6. AT LEAST CONSIDER ADOPTION.

You owe it to yourself and to your child not to close your mind to adoption as you look into the best possible decision for your life and the life of the baby. If you are afraid of losing your child, remember that open adoption practices allow you to see your child and have ongoing contact for the rest of your life. As a birth mother, you have the right to a great deal of control over whom you choose to parent your child.

7. START TALKING TO GOD.

God knows all about your situation and loves you more than you can imagine. He doesn't see that you have ruined your life. He sees you as his favorite child. He loves you enough never to turn his back on you.

When you begin to feel depressed and guilty, remember this verse: "We set our hearts at rest in his presence whenever our hearts condemn us. For God is greater than our hearts, and he knows everything" (1 John 3:19–20).

God has been through this before. He helped arrange

some very famous adoptions in the Bible: Moses, Samuel, and Esther were all adopted, and Moses and Samuel were both "open adoption" cases. Read about them. They might give you some idea of how much love God had for their mothers to provide for them so well.

PART II
Abortion

The Abortion Option

"Get rid of it quickly!" "No one ever has to know."

Do you really want to have an abortion, or is someone pressuring you with statements like these? In a state of crisis it is difficult to think clearly. We tend to allow others to make our decisions for us. We give up our responsibility to ourselves by listening to others and allowing them to influence us into making decisions we may not have made otherwise. That's partly how you got pregnant. That's partly what is causing you to consider abortion.

After reading the decisions of the girls in this section and the adoption section, you can begin to see that there was someone nearby encouraging them in that particular decision. A close family member or friend stood by suggesting that they either have the child and place it for adoption or have an abortion.

Ultimately, each decision you make is yours alone. And the aftereffects are yours alone, affecting only you, not the others who want to influence your decision. Deep in your heart, you know what decision you want to make if you are pregnant.

Most people have no idea of the physical, emotional, and spiritual aftereffects of abortion. Everyone reacts differently. As you read the stories of the three women in this section, you will notice some similarities and differences in their reactions to abortion.

One of the women interviewed claims the abortion didn't affect her at all. In fact, she said it made her more responsible. The truth is, she was badly hurt by her boyfriend, who agreed to pay for the abortion but had little to do with her after that. Since then, she has chosen to date guys that use her, escaping into the wild nightlife of California to numb her pain rather than dealing with her critically damaged self-image.

Two of the women interviewed later attempted suicide. Their prolonged grief and self-hatred over terminating the pregnancy almost took their lives. Only after much counseling and finding healing in a relationship with Jesus Christ were these women set free of the aftermath of abortion.

The decision to have an abortion is a major decision. The worst part about decision making in the case of an unplanned pregnancy is that it has to be done in the middle of one's first major crisis in life. Teenage pregnancy is a traumatic experience, and rarely are good decisions made during times of great emotional upheaval.

Any decision on what to do with an unwanted pregnancy is going to be painful to make. But the aftereffects do not have to ruin your life forever. Healing begins with talking over the decision with others and obtaining all the facts of each option. Going into any decision with your eyes wide open will prepare you for the aftereffects. Then, in the aftermath, talking about your feelings and thoughts with others, expressing the grief and anger, will defuse problems that could arise.

Believe it or not, an unplanned pregnancy can be a catalyst for positive change in your life. The pregnancy doesn't have to doom you to a life of hidden guilt and grief, nor does it have to alienate you from your family, especially if you deal with the situation together, as a family. Through this experience you will definitely gain a more realistic view of life. You will discover decision-making skills you didn't know you had. You will acknowledge your strengths as well as your weaknesses. And you will discover that you *can* make it through a crisis.

PROS AND CONS

The spiritual, physical, and emotional effects of abortion are outlined in the "Abortion: Questions to Ask Yourself" chapter at the end of this section. If you are considering having an abortion, consider what you are about to do to your body. Abortion isn't always going to hide the problem pregnancy.

TYPES OF ABORTION

Several types of abortion procedures are available. They are performed according to how many weeks pregnant you are. A successful abortion removes all of the contents of the uterus including the fetus (or embryo, as it is called in its first two months of life), the placenta, which nourishes the fetus until delivery, and the built-up lining of the uterus.

The most common abortion is done during the first three months of pregnancy and is called "vacuum aspiration" or "suction." The procedure is performed in a clinic or doctor's office. The girl's cervix is numbed and dilated so that a plastic tube can be inserted through the cervix and into the uterus. The other end of the tube contains a suction pump that breaks up and removes the developing fetus and surrounding matter. It has a low risk of infection and, if done properly, a low risk of damaging the uterus by tearing the lining.

A "D & C" (dilation and curettage) is used in pregnancies from two to four months old. The girl is put to sleep and, after dilating the cervix, the lining of the uterus is scraped with a spoon-shaped instrument called a curette. This is riskier because the chances of infection and bleeding are greater. Also, some women react adversely to the effects of anesthesia.

During the fourth through sixth months of pregnancy a combination of the vacuum aspiration and the D & C are used. The procedure is called a "D & E" (dilation and evacuation). This requires an overnight hospital stay as the cervix must be dilated wider than required earlier in the pregnancy. By this time, the fetus is more fully developed, and it requires more extensive work to remove it. Injections of saline or other solutions into the amniotic sac surrounding the fetus cut off its life support and burn the fetus until it expires. The injections cause the girl to have contractions as if she is delivering a baby, and the fetus is expelled through the cervix. Sometimes the placenta doesn't come out and the doctor has to perform a D & C, requiring a longer hospital stay. It's a lot like going through labor and delivery, but there is nothing to show for the trauma involved.

Abortions are rarely performed during the last three months of pregnancy. By the time of the third trimester (six months), almost every fetus is capable of living outside the mother's womb with limited medical support. Yet it is legal in some states to have an abortion even at this late stage. The procedure used is like a caesarean section. A small cut is made in the abdomen to remove the fetus. This procedure is also used if a woman cannot use any of the above methods for health reasons. However, it is riskier than the other procedures. Late-pregnancy abortions can result in the baby being born alive and having health complications due to its premature birth. Emotional trauma to the mother would be much greater in this case.

A lot of things are said about the aftereffects of abortion on a woman's body. The fact is, one abortion probably will not affect a woman's chances of having children in later years. Multiple abortions will most likely cause damage to a woman's uterus and give her problems later in life.

Abortion is not a method of birth control. It is an operation. Birth control prevents pregnancy; it doesn't terminate it. If you are sexually active and not on a form of birth control you are playing games with your physical and emotional health. Read about the girls in this section and consider how serious the "game" can be. Having sex without birth control is like playing Russian roulette. Somebody is going to get hurt. And that somebody will be you.

It Only Takes
Three Minutes

No one ever realizes that the aftereffects of abortion can be really traumatic. Feelings of guilt and thoughts of being dirty and unlovable can overwhelm the woman who has had an abortion. For Anita, severe depression overshadowed her for three years before she sought healing in a relationship with God. Today, the effects of her past lie behind her.

A veteran of many relationships, Anita believes the abortion she had as a junior in high school affected her relationships with her boyfriends for years afterward. Her story has a particular twist to it. She was a Christian at the time she became pregnant and decided to terminate the pregnancy through abortion to "cover her sin." The spiritual struggles over guilt and condemnation haunted her for years. The fact that she was outspokenly anti-abortion and yet opted for an abortion intensified her guilt and shame.

At first glance you would think Anita was an artist from London. Her giant designer earrings and sophisticated clothes look as if they were bought in a suave London boutique. Bangs stiffened by hair spray curl in a four-inch wave over her head. The streak of flair to her dress and her slow, steady walk cause heads to turn and people to notice her. When she speaks, every word is deliberately chosen as if she is measuring its effect on the listener. Her style creates an air of knowing more than a twenty-three-year-old Southern Californian should know.

"I'll tell you how I met this guy and what happened between us," Anita began nervously, her hand plucking strands of grass from the lawn on which we sat. "I went to Europe when I was a junior in high school. The chaperones gave us a lot of freedom, a lot more freedom than I had at home. We would go out on the town, drink, and party as much as we wanted to. It was acceptable over there. They had no drinking age. One night in Germany, I met this guy from Holland. He was staying at the same youth hostel we were in. It was like our eyes met across the room and connected right away. Instant wow! So I went out with him while I was there."

Away from home, Anita for the first time experienced boundless freedom: no parents on the lookout, and plenty of people to party with. Anita decided to leave her Christianity at home and party with the rest of the group. Kids who wouldn't drink at home felt a sense of adventure in being abroad. Kids who wouldn't pair up at home suddenly found themselves drunk and having sex in someone's hotel room. Anita decided that she would party with the group but vetoed sleeping with any of the guys. Until Carl.

"It was so spontaneous," Anita explained. "We were alone and he asked me if I wanted to sleep with him. I said, 'No, I can't, because I am a Christian and I don't believe in premarital sex.' I started telling him about my belief in God and he replied that he didn't believe the same way but if that was how I felt we wouldn't sleep together. So we started talking about other things and all of a sudden I said, 'OK, I will.'"

In a split second, Anita chose to give in. After all, she was on vacation, and part of the adventure was having sex with a stranger from Holland. Beliefs were something you left back home, not some extra baggage to haul around on vacation—especially if you pick up your beliefs from your family rather than understanding them for yourself. She felt like she wanted to explore another side of life and grow up.

Within a couple of weeks, the party was over and the European travelers returned home. Anita knew she was pregnant about two weeks later when morning sickness assaulted her stomach. It dawned on her that this was going to be more than a simple case of the flu. She consulted her friends at school, who advised her to get an abortion. A short visit to a crisis pregnancy clinic confirmed that she was pregnant. Confusion clouded her thoughts. Reeling from the shock of being told that she, an outspoken Christian on campus who condemned abortion and premarital sex, had gotten caught, Anita heard little the counselor said. Something about going to a doctor regularly if she was going to keep her baby and her body changing for the rest of her life stuck in her memory. The counselor asked questions like "How are you going to support this baby?" to jar her into thinking abortion was the best option for her.

When Anita talked to her counselor about God, she said, "God's not going to do anything. He'll forgive you if that's your issue. Really, it's not wrong because the fetus isn't human. You're six weeks pregnant and you need to make a decision now." The clinic's message, loud and clear, was that if Anita wanted to keep her baby then something must be wrong with her. Anita went home to think about her options.

Later that day, Carl, the guy from Holland, called to surprise her. Anita couldn't bring herself to tell him that she was pregnant but burst into tears as she was talking to him. He thought she missed him terribly and was crying because she was so glad to hear from him. He never knew that Anita was pregnant from the night they spent together. He never had the opportunity to participate in deciding the fate of his unborn child.

Anita felt like she couldn't tell her parents because sex was never talked about except at church when the priest repeated that sex before marriage was a sin. The vibes at home led Anita to believe that sex was bad.

Anita couldn't look for much support at school either. Since she was a more vocal Christian on campus, she had a reputation of being a good girl. She was judgmental about people who slept around and had abortions— until it happened to her. Then she thought, *Wow, I'm one of these people.* She wanted to hide the fact that she had sex before marriage, and so she decided to have an abortion—even though she knew it was wrong.

Anita didn't know what to expect when she arrived at the abortion clinic. "It only takes three minutes," was all her counselor told her. No explanation of the procedure itself or how it would feel was given to her. And she was too afraid to ask. Or maybe she was still in shock over the realization that she was pregnant. For Anita, the experience bordered on terror.

She walked into the clinic waiting room. Inside, women ranging in age from twelve to thirty-eight years old waited anxiously. Every five minutes Anita could hear the whir of the suction machine and the crying of a woman.

Finally a nurse took Anita into a side room and asked her to put on a gown. Then she took a blood sample and told Anita to wait for the doctor.

Anita sat alone in the room, listening to the vacuuming noise of the suction machine. *Be strong,* she told herself. She knew that she could walk out of there at any minute . . . but she just couldn't move.

Two women walked into the room where Anita sat waiting. One of the ladies was there to hold Anita's hand and comfort her during the operation. The other woman was a doctor. They told her to lay back on the table.

Anita broke down and started crying in front of them. They looked at her strangely. The lady who was along for moral support said, "What's wrong with you? Who told you about the procedure for terminating a pregnancy? Has someone been telling you this is wrong? It's no big deal. It only takes about three minutes and that's it. Three minutes and it's over. Why are you crying?"

She cried so hard that she couldn't talk. But she wanted to scream at them, "Can't you see what I'm doing? Don't you see this is a sin? Don't you see that I am murdering my baby?" But they were clueless. All they said was "What's wrong with you? It only takes three minutes."

The three minutes passed and it was over. The changes that had begun in her body as it prepared itself to nourish the fetus were abruptly halted as the abortion was completed. Anita felt that whoever had been growing inside of her before the abortion had been cut off, torn out of her. And her body reversed its course of preparations.

The women took her to a recovery room, where Anita lay for about an hour before dressing and leaving for home. As she lay there, the aftereffects of abortion settled on her. She began to stuff her grief deep into the pockets of her mind.

Experiencing an abortion is to undergo voluntary physical trauma. Your system goes into shock. Anita said it felt like something was ripped out of her; she sensed the physical trauma to her body. Following an abortion, a time of bleeding may last a day or longer. For a couple of weeks afterward, Anita was told not to pick up any heavy objects or do any strenuous activities. Otherwise, the bleeding could become severe. Instead of following doctor's orders, Anita went back to work unloading crates of eggs and stacking them in the family store. During the next three days, she began feeling weaker and started hemorrhaging. She ran a fever and told her mother that it was just another one of her really bad periods.

Anita told me, "I remember my mother walking into my bedroom, and I wanted to tell her so badly what had happened. But I couldn't. I didn't want anyone to know. I knew that if I was that sick by the following day I was going to have to go back to the clinic or into a hospital emergency room to stop the bleeding. I prayed that night and said, 'God, I don't want this to come into the open. Please keep me from dying or having to go back to that doctor. Please help me hide this experience.' The next day I was fine. The bleeding had stopped. I think God had a lot of mercy on me and healed me."

When your body is in a state of trauma, it affects your emotions and your thoughts. In other words, you become stressed out. Some women who have abortions breeze through the experience, and it never seems to affect them later in life. Others add an abortion experience to a list of other traumatic episodes in their life and have a hard time coping with anything later on. Everyone reacts differently. But everyone needs someone to hold them, listen to them, and comfort them after a traumatic experience involving death or loss. Your emotions get all tangled up inside of you, and talking helps untangle them. But few people know how to start talking or even how they feel during a time like this. They don't think others will understand. Anita desperately needed someone to talk to, but it was a few years later before she finally had an opportunity to talk, to untangle all of the emotional pain she had stuffed inside.

Anita found it difficult to live with herself after the abortion. She felt like she had defiled herself and was no longer fit for marriage. She thought she would never be able to have children after the procedure was over. She felt like a murderer. She believed that if she did have children they would be retarded or would have birth defects because she had committed this great sin. Guilt and fear began to gnaw at her. At that point, she started destroying herself.

For a time, she went on with school, attending a Bible college with some of her friends after high school. She started dating guys who couldn't care less about her. Eventually, she fell in love with a guy named George. They were both in college, and he was on his way to becoming a pro tennis player. For a while their relationship was going so well that they got engaged.

One day, out of the blue, George broke the engagement with a flurry of rude words, trying to blame Anita for being unlovable. The truth was, he was more interested in a tennis career than marriage.

"It was devastating," Anita said, remembering. "I raged at God: 'See God? I've been telling you how I am. I've been telling you that I'm dirty—that I'm a whore and a murderer. Everybody's seen it in me!' All the subconscious thoughts about being a murderer came out when George broke up with me. And I believed these thoughts."

Anita went into a rage, throwing everything she could lay her hands on, tearing up every picture of George she could find. She was so furious with George that she wanted to kill him. Instead, she tried to kill herself.

Anita swallowed a handful of pills and lay back on her bed. Within a few minutes shooting pains began darting through her head. Suddenly, she realized that she didn't want to die and called a friend who came over with her mother and called the paramedics. The hospital kept her on the mental ward for three days of observation and evaluation by a psychiatrist. For Anita, talking with the psychiatrist helped her put things in perspective. The psychiatrist listened to Anita's story, then told her that she was not a bad person, not a murderer, nor any of the negative things she thought she was because of what she'd done or what had been done to her by others.

For three years after the abortion Anita lived in depression. There were days when she couldn't get up in the morning. She would suffer anxiety attacks or get really angry for no reason at all. Now, five years after the experience, she believes the depression lifted partially during talks with a counselor and partially because she became involved with a young adults group at her church who love her for who she is.

In the last couple of years, Anita has allowed God to draw closer and walk through more healing with her. It's not like God sprinkled magic dust on her head to make her okay. There are a lot of old tapes still playing in her head that create momentary feelings of guilt and sadness. But when they start to play, she remembers that God has forgiven her for every sin ever done in her life and will never hold it against her. She also recalls two supernatural experiences that brought great healing into her life, releasing her from the guilt and pain of the abortion.

"Once in a dream, I saw Jesus holding my baby. It was a little girl. When I saw her in the arms of Jesus, love poured from me, and I had to ask her forgiveness for my own sake. She seemed to say, 'Mom, I forgive you. I love you.' And I was able to tell her that I love her. That was a really healing experience.

"Another time when others were praying for me I saw myself in the clinic waiting for my abortion. Jesus stood at the foot of the bed crying. He was bawling just as hard as I was. He hurt so badly for me, crying tears of compassion even in the midst of my sin. God really showed me that he is understanding of why I do what I do. Not that it's right. But he knows when I've been programmed to think certain ways and react certain ways. It's his job to know!

"God and I worked together for my healing, because I allowed him to draw near. I've allowed him to expose the lies and defenses that I've lived under, like self-judgment, self-hatred, and feelings of worthlessness. He gave me a new set of tools to work with, new ways of reacting and combating guilt, to live a healthy way. First he had to tell me the truth about how he saw me—that he wasn't a God who pointed his finger at me and damned me to hell for what I did. Instead, he was a God who was hurting because I was hurting."

A Twinge of Conscience

College was a new experience in freedom for Ann. Raised in a traditional, all-American family, the world's problems passed by only on the evening news. Her neighborhood and her life were sheltered from most of society's ills like divorce, drugs, gangs, teen pregnancy, and suicides. Life was fun and simple—for a while.

By the end of her freshman year in college, Ann was faced with a decision which would affect her outlook on life for years to come. She was no longer a kid playing in the neighborhood, heedless of the repercussions from her actions. Ann discovered that sex is not a toy you could put away after you were through playing with it. Seemingly overnight, Ann grew up.

In the typical American family, sex is not brought up at the dinner table. Parents realize that daughters and sons are suddenly entering into adolescence, but they hope to delay that sex education talk for another year or so. By then, the kids have picked up more knowledge than their parents were ever prepared to tell. And there is nothing left to discuss. Or so they think.

Ann came from one of these families. As she said, "My sex ed talk from my mother came when I was about thirteen years old. She said, 'Do you know everything?' And my sister and I said yes. She said, 'Do you have any questions?' And we said no. That was it. I learned everything from my friends."

School wasn't much help either. She went to junior high in New Jersey, and in high school, her family moved to Texas. In the school system back East, sex education wasn't taught. In Texas, sex education was taught among friends.

"I remember when my friend first told me about how

men and women do it," Ann said. "I was probably about eleven. I truly thought sex was the way you see it in movies. But sex wasn't like I expected. I was a virgin right up until I was a freshman in college. Sex came as a rude awakening. It wasn't like it is in the movies at all."

In college, Ann met a senior, and they went out a couple of times during her first year in college. Just before he graduated he caught a dose of the "Let's do what we can before I leave" syndrome. Ann gave in. A few weeks before graduation they spent the night together. He graduated and left town with no promises of a lasting relationship and no ideas of keeping in touch. After all, their evening together meant nothing. It was just a night of fun.

Within a month, Ann realized her period had not come on schedule. The night of fun was beginning to feel like a night of regret. "At the time I was in total denial. I thought, *No way. No way.* I told my roommate that I didn't get my period and she said, 'You better get checked.' They didn't have home pregnancy tests around, so I had to go in for a test. I remember thinking that if I didn't get my period that week then I would be about six weeks pregnant. So I went to Planned Parenthood and they told me to bring back a urine sample in the morning. Well, I put it in the wrong type of container. So there I was sweating it out, waiting to find out what the test result was, and they couldn't draw conclusive results. So I had to go in the next day, and then they told me that I was definitely pregnant."

Ann sat there while the counselor was talking, thinking over and over again, *I can't believe this. This isn't happening to me.* She was totally shocked. This sort of thing never happened to the all-American family. In her mind, only lower-class Americans got caught doing such things.

Ann immediately knew what she was going to do. "There really was no debate. I knew right away that I

A Twinge of Conscience

was going to have to get an abortion. I was in college intending to get a degree. If I had the child I would have to move back home with my parents and get a minimum wage job. I knew having a baby would have completely ended any type of progress. So I knew in the long run it was the best thing."

When the counselor informed Ann that she was pregnant, she asked Ann what she would like to do about it. Ann replied, "I really have no choice but to get an abortion." Just like that, abruptly and decisively, Ann made her choice. She was getting it done and she didn't want to talk about it. Case closed. The woman told her about the procedure and suggested they talk about contraception afterward, during a follow-up counseling session.

When Ann decided to schedule the abortion she called the guy she had slept with and asked him to pay for half of the abortion. Totally shocked, he agreed nevertheless. Ann said, "He was as nice as someone whom you don't have a relationship with, which we didn't. After the guy found out I was going to get an abortion, he didn't treat me very well. He called me the day that I went in, but I never heard from him again, ever. He called me that day and that was it. I think I lost a little respect for guys after that. The majority of guys have it easy. They say, 'Oh well, I'll pay for half of it,' but paying is all they have to do. They're not the ones on the table."

A friend of Ann's agreed to drive her to the clinic and go in with her. "It was a whole lot worse than anyone ever told me it would be or I ever thought it would be," Ann remembered. "They explain the procedure, but they don't tell you how it will feel. They give you the choice whether you want to be knocked out or just have the pelvic area numbed by local anesthesia so you can't feel much. I went with a local, and it felt awful. The actual procedure hurt. It seemed like it took forever, but

I guess it was only a three-minute procedure. While I was in there, I heard another girl totally freaking out. It was scary, man!

"But I will never, ever forget the feeling I had when it was all over and everybody cleared the room and they told me to get dressed. I felt like dirt. I felt like the lowest thing. I went through a grieving process right then, feeling very alone. I was devastated emotionally because stuff like this didn't happen to me or to any of my friends. It wasn't until after I started opening up about it that I found out how many people have had abortions. I couldn't believe the number of my friends who had abortions and kept it private. Sure, you heard rumors about abortions in school, but I couldn't believe that something like that had happened to me.

"Having the abortion taught me that there are definite consequences for our actions. This was the first time in my life that I had to answer for anything. And you have to make a choice, you know."

If Ann had known she would get pregnant from a one-night stand she would never have had sex in the first place. The decision against bringing a child into the world, against paying the consequences of quick actions, begins with the decision not to have sex. Once life begins, it is not ours to take.

The night before Ann went into the clinic she started to realize that the decision to have an abortion was not as easy as she'd thought. She had always loved children and felt like she would have been the last person in the world to harm a child. Ann felt a twinge of conscience when it dawned on her that this abortion would terminate the life of another human being. She called a really good friend who had been in school with her but moved away. Ann asked her what she thought about abortion and she said, "Look. Go back and read some of our biology books and resign yourself to the fact that it is

A Twinge of Conscience

a fetus. It isn't a baby." She went through all the medical justifications of abortion.

"It was a little bit of a comfort to me," Ann recalled, "but you can't go into an abortion without thinking you are killing someone. You just settle it in your own mind. In my conscience, I felt like it was early enough. It wasn't a life. I had it done because I loved children, and I didn't think it fair for the child to grow up without a father and with a limited future."

Even as Ann spoke, I could hear the wondering in her voice. The fact that she wondered if she was killing someone should have indicated that her conscience was trying to tell her something. A conscience is like a little warning bell that sounds when you are about to do something wrong. A conscience tries to tell you when you are about to mess things up. Ann felt that same twinge of conscience when she gave in and had sex with her boyfriend. But she did it despite thinking that it was wrong.

"It took about four months before I started realizing that I didn't depend on anybody to get me through this emotionally afterward. I didn't rely on God. I didn't rely on family—I didn't even tell my family. To this day they do not know. I had a real fear of them being judgmental. But my friends helped me out. My roommate lent me the other half of the money. Still, I feel as though nobody helped me out of this thing but me. I got through it and I'm a much stronger person for it."

Although Ann felt like she went through the abortion alone, she had three very close friends who helped her go through the days immediately following the abortion. Two of her friends had had an abortion in the past. They had told Ann about it when they were first becoming friends, so Ann felt free to tell them she was considering an abortion and allowed them to comfort her afterward. But even with their help, Ann felt different, isolated. Her friends hadn't grown up in a middle-class family where nothing bad ever happened. So when they got pregnant, they weren't nearly as shocked or devastated as Ann.

Ann's friends threw her a party when she arrived home from the clinic. They stocked up on munchies and movies and set up a fun evening so that Ann could put the whole experience out of her mind and get on with life.

Abortion was the perfect out for Ann. No one would have to know and life could go on as planned. It would be Ann's secret. But secrets are funny things. They won't stay locked up in a cage called memories. Instead, they run along your nerve endings and cause you to feel tense and alone. Then they unlock another cage filled with emotions and turn them loose. Guilt, fear, and anger shoot up your nerves. Pretty soon, these hidden secrets and rampant emotions start planting funny thoughts in your mind and cause you to act differently. Ann's secrets made her act tougher. She began thinking she didn't need anyone else in this world and could rely on herself alone. She kept dating guys who treated her like an object rather than a person.

Ann said, "I think that guys try real hard in college to get girls in the sack and don't ever think beyond that. And girls don't either until they live through a pregnancy. But guys *never* think beyond. If they were the ones that got pregnant, then they would have to start thinking. I still enjoy guys and have a lot of guy friends, but my favorite saying is, 'Men are pigs'—especially the guys I've gone out with since then."

The hurt Ann felt from going through the experience alone, without the "father" of the baby caring about what she went through, lingers on even today. Almost six years after the abortion, her relationships with men still suffer. She looks for love in all the wrong places, attracting all the wrong guys. She believes the abortion experience made her more responsible and a stronger

A Twinge of Conscience

person. However, her life today is filled with nights on the dance floor and nights spent drinking with friends, telling each other tales of what they did the night before under the influence of too much alcohol.

People who rely on drugs or alcohol (even for "fun") are seeking to numb their pain, drown their rampant emotions, and wash away their secrets. Strong and responsible people don't act that way. Strong people are those who listen to that twinge of conscience telling them to stop and think before they act. Strong people are those who can ask for help rather than hide a problem.

What Am I Doing?

As Ann's story shows, emotional healing from the aftermath of abortion takes a long time. Guilt feelings may lead to self-destructive attempts to numb the pain. Some women begin to drink or use drugs. Others may suddenly become promiscuous, sleeping or flirting with every guy that catches their eye. Suicidal thoughts and actions can occur years after such a traumatic experience as having an abortion. By then, the pain is seen as an enemy to be destroyed rather than the key to unlocking a new self, and the abortion may seem like a nightmare from the past. But its memory lurks in the subconscious and creates a confusing tangle of emotional pain and guilt.

Rita grew up spoiled and ignored by her wealthy Argentinian family. She was eighteen years old when she learned that she was pregnant. Pressured into having an abortion by her boyfriend and mother, Rita lashed out in the aftermath of the abortion in self-destructive ways. For many years afterward, her abortion impacted her with feelings of guilt, self-destructive behavior, and struggles in marriage and future motherhood. But Rita has received much healing over the years, some of it directly related to the abortion she had as a teenager.

Rita's story is common to many girls raised in wealthy homes. In a country where abortion is illegal, family money bought the doctor who performed the abortion so that the "good name" of the family might be preserved by sweeping the whole affair under the rug. Having sex before marriage was tolerable. However, getting caught was a cardinal sin and brought shame to the family.

Rita's boyfriend had pressured her for a whole year to have sex. "It was hard for me to decide to give in to a physical relationship. But I was really in love with this guy," Rita explained. "So after a year, we started having sex, and within a few months I was pregnant. He was using protection, but it was a time when I said I still had my period and there was no danger of getting pregnant."

Little did Rita know that a woman can get pregnant at any time of the month. And women can conceive even when they are using birth control pills and other forms of contraceptives. You receive a lot of misinformation from the media. Safe sex is a myth. The safest sex is no sex at all. Even if the guy is using protection in the form of a condom, there is no guarantee that pregnancy or sexually transmitted diseases will be prevented.

Noticing the interruption in Rita's monthly cycle, her mother sent her to the family doctor, who gave her a shot of hormones. Her period still didn't come. Finally, Rita returned to the doctor, an older man who had taken care of her mother and her grandmother. The doctor ran a few tests and refused to tell her the results. He was embarrassed. After all, Rita came from a very wealthy, proper family who lived in a predominately Catholic country. Such matters as pregnancy out of wedlock were shameful to mention.

Rita and her boyfriend finally decided that she must be pregnant and arranged to have a pregnancy test done elsewhere. Her boyfriend took her specimen to the lab and promised to call her with the results.

Finally he called. "No, you're not pregnant," he said, "but I am going to come over tonight." So he came over and took Rita for a drive. And then he told her she really was pregnant.

"I was so happy," Rita said. "I kept telling him, 'I can't believe I'm carrying your child.' I was really in love with this guy. But he started saying right away, 'I don't think we should have this child. I need to finish my studies. We're too young. I don't want it to live without its parents. I really don't think we should have this child.'"

Despair gripped Rita. Giving up hope that her boyfriend would change his mind, she turned to her mother for help. One day, while her mother was soaking in the bathtub, Rita went in and said, "Mom, I need to tell you something."

"What is it?"

"I'm pregnant."

"I can still see her face when I told her I was pregnant," Rita recalled. "I mean, she didn't even think I could have sex. Her first response was gasping in total panic, 'Oh! What am I going to tell my friends?'"

Angered that her mother cared more about her friends than about her, Rita began to shut her mother out of her life. She saw that her mother's reputation in the community and climbing the social ladder was more important to her than her own family. Rita's father never mentioned that he even knew of the pregnancy. He ignored the situation. "That was the secret message in our home," Rita explained. "Whenever there are problems, you keep quiet. Nobody wants to know. Everything needs to be perfect and if there are any problems, we don't want to know about it. So you keep it to yourself."

Rita's mother began to pressure her to follow her boyfriend's advice and have an abortion. She thought that an abortion would eliminate the problem and make everything return to normal.

When you are in a crisis and no one in the family wants to talk about the situation, you feel like you are caught in a crazy whirlwind that no one else sees. What you don't realize is that everyone else is caught up in their own emotional whirlwind and all they can see is their own problem. They are so blown about that they don't even know they are in the middle of a storm. That's when others can help. If Rita had called a crisis pregnancy counselor she would have had the emotional support she needed. Instead, she stood in the storm alone, eventually drifting the way of the loudest voice.

Rita kept to herself. Her anger turned inward,

twisting her reactions and pushing her toward self-destruction. For hours she sat alone in her room, rocking back and forth, singing lullabies and writing poems to the unborn child. In those few weeks Rita fell in love with the baby beginning to grow in her womb. She felt like she wasn't alone. But she knew she wouldn't be allowed to keep the baby.

Eventually, her mother teamed up with her boyfriend to confront her with the news that she was to have an abortion and to have one quickly. "They both stood over me pointing with accusing fingers and saying, 'You have to do this. You have to have an abortion.' They said that this was the only solution possible for the baby."

Rita knew that if she had the baby she couldn't go on living with her parents, nor could she go with her boyfriend to his college. She knew she would have ended up living in a small apartment, working to pay for expenses, then having to pay someone to look after her child. "What kind of a life did I have to offer him?" Rita asked. "He wouldn't even know me because I'd be out working all day. And I was totally spoiled. I didn't even know what working was—it was a totally foreign concept in my mind. So I thought, for the sake of my baby, I won't have him. I couldn't perceive giving such conditions to my child. It was like sacrificing him for his own benefit. That was the argument I needed in order to go ahead and do it. I couldn't grab onto anything else to convince myself to have the abortion."

Caught between her own conscious desire to have the baby and the force of the two most significant people in her life arguing in one loud voice against teenage motherhood, Rita decided to have an abortion. Her mother's shame would be covered up so that none of her friends would ever know. Her boyfriend could continue his education and plans for his life without further responsibilities. And Rita?

Well, her anger against her mother was now fueled by

more anger against her boyfriend for not intervening and allowing her to have the baby. She couldn't forgive her boyfriend for what she perceived as "taking my baby away." Her love turned to resentment, and their relationship grew more distant. It seemed as if one day they were in love, passionately involved and on their way to happily-ever-after-land. Then, just as suddenly, they turned against each other.

True love does not demand its own way. If your boyfriend or parents pressure you to make a decision that goes against your conscience, that is not love. They are seeking their own best interest, not yours. Sometimes, total strangers offering advice and assistance demonstrate the truest love.

Not only did Rita not want to have an abortion, obtaining one proved to be difficult. In Argentina, abortion is illegal. There are no abortion clinics, and doctors willing to "do the favor" were secretive about their practice, performing abortions in their offices under the guise of routine gynecological care. Midwives, women who assisted in births at home, also performed abortions for those who could not find a willing doctor or those who could not afford a doctor. Because they lacked medical knowledge and instruments, these midwives often caused harm to those desperate enough to come to them for an abortion. Rita explained, "Often the news would report on a midwife caught doing an abortion. Sometimes women did horrible things to themselves to try to have an abortion. I remember two or three incidents when my maids got real sick and my parents ran them to the hospital because they were hemorrhaging. I bet you they were trying to abort their babies."

Self-induced abortions rarely work, however. Jumping up and down, causing trauma to your stomach, trying to remove the fetus by force, or taking an overdose of pills will only result in harm to yourself. In

79

the early stages of pregnancy, the mother's body forms an incredible protective system to shield the fetus from harm. Trying to remove or destroy that life before it's ready to be born will only harm your body. Sometimes, that harm is beyond repair. Those who try self-induced abortions to hide their pregnancy usually wind up in the hospital for all to see.

Rita's boyfriend found a doctor willing to perform the secret abortion in his office. They purchased the anesthesia and brought it with them for the scheduled abortion. (The doctor could have come under suspicion by the police by buying inordinate amounts of anesthesia for his office.) The procedure itself went quickly. Rita remembered being semi-unconscious, but she was not told how the abortion would be performed. She didn't even know what method the doctor used.

Rita recalled, "My boyfriend brought me back home afterward. I walked into the house and went upstairs to bed. My mom sent the maid upstairs with a bowl of soup for me. She was playing bridge with her friends downstairs and couldn't be bothered. So she sent something for me to drink, and that was it. She never talked about it again."

The silence within the house became an echo chamber for Rita's thoughts and caused her anger to grow. She would walk by her mother and sneer that she was having sex with her boyfriend again. "I became almost sadistic as I tried to hurt her. I really went into crisis and was mentally sick after the abortion. I would scratch things and couldn't stop, or I would comb my hair compulsively. I'd burst into hysteria, start screaming, screaming, screaming.

"I would cry a lot and tell my boyfriend that I was going to kill myself because I didn't want to live like this. Finally, I was sitting on my dad's side of the bed, and I knew he had a gun in his night table. I was suicidal. My boyfriend and my mom were there. I took out the gun and put it up to my head. When my mom saw that, she got really scared and said, 'We'll send you to a psychiatrist.' That was what I wanted. I needed help. My father was against it because he thought people would say, 'Oh, look at his daughter. She's crazy.' I said, 'Dad, going to a psychiatrist doesn't make me crazy.' I wanted to say, 'You make me crazy,' but I didn't." With the help of a psychologist, Rita began to sort through her emotions and ceased her self-destructive acts.

Many families are like Rita's, refusing to confront a problem and work through it together. Instead, they send a secret message to each other, "Don't talk to anybody about your problems. Don't trust anybody. Push down those emotions and pretend like you don't feel anything." But they are asking you to do the impossible. Keeping silent about problems at home is like blowing too much air into a balloon. Sooner or later, it's going to explode.

A normal, healthy human being needs to talk about her problems. A normal, healthy human being needs to express her emotions. If your family refuses to acknowledge those needs, you must talk to other people who can help, like pastors, psychologists, and counselors. These people won't ask you to suppress your thoughts and emotions. Instead, they will help you sort through them, standing by you as you express your pain, anger, and guilt.

After a period of time in counseling, Rita broke off the relationship with her boyfriend, met an American, married him, and moved to the United States. She miscarried their first child, a process called "spontaneous abortion."

Eventually, she and her husband had their first daughter. Rita described her feelings about her new daughter. "I just couldn't love her. I couldn't even breast-feed her. It was very hard. I would put her to my breast and no milk would come out. I would go into the bathroom and the milk would flow out of my breast. But when she was at the breast, nothing. It was an emotional connection. I couldn't give her any affection due to a vow that I had made. I had told myself after the abortion that I couldn't love another child. With the second baby it was a little bit better. Then I got divorced two months later."

By this time, Rita had not only lost two unborn children but a husband as well. It took many years for her to release the pain she felt over these losses. She returned to Argentina and began to seek greater healing. It wasn't long before she found someone who could lift the guilt from her and replace it with the love she had always sought. Rita met an American couple who began to tell her about Jesus Christ. "When I came to know the Lord, right away I started feeling Christ's healing love for me, no strings attached, no matter what. I never sensed any condemnation from anybody. Every time I shared my abortion experience with someone, their response was loving."

Rita was discovering a new kind of love—a love that is patient and kind, never jealous or envious, never boastful or proud, never haughty or selfish or rude. She asked Jesus to reveal his love for her and he did, showing his acceptance through others.

During the healing process, she went to a conference where a woman named Judith McNutt was to speak. Suddenly, while the woman was speaking, Rita had a vivid daydream that lifted the remaining grief from her. "I saw a picture of two blond boys with long white nightgowns jumping and playing on feather beds. They were very happy. All at once Jesus came in and said (now I didn't even realize this), 'I know that the biggest pain that you carry is that you are unable to take care of your children that you have with you, but there are two that you cannot take care of, and you don't know how they are doing. I wanted you to see that they are with me, well cared for, and happy.'"

Rita was greatly comforted by the vision. She had the feeling that when she got to heaven, her two unborn children would run to her, and she would get to know them. Christ knows that a mother is always concerned about the welfare of her children. So he showed Rita that her sons were doing well—because they were with him.

Abortion: Questions to Ask Yourself

I care too much about you to recommend that you have an abortion. Even though any unplanned pregnancy is traumatic, I believe that those who have abortions face a greater inner struggle than those who place a child for adoption or decide to raise their child. The spiritual, physical, and emotional effects of abortion are damaging in the long run. Before you make that final decision to have an abortion, please take a moment to ask yourself these questions.

1. WHOSE PLAN ARE YOU FOLLOWING?

You probably know all of the arguments for and against abortion. The spiritual arguments against abortion are not often voiced. Some of these reasons are not even known because God hasn't fully revealed all of the mysteries of life to us. But I want to give you something to consider.

When you were conceived, God knew who you were and everything that would happen to you in your life. He desired that you would come to know him and the love he has for you. All of the plans he has for your life were written down for you before you were born. Yet he knew that there is a very real spiritual enemy named Satan who would try to rob you of the love God has for you and kill any possible interaction with this loving God. Satan is also known as the Destroyer, one who seeks to destroy lives before they are born or even after they have lived on this earth for a time.

So there are two plans afoot. God's plan is for you to come to know his love for you and what you are here on earth for. Satan's plan is to bring as much destruction into your life as possible to keep you from God.

You are not here by accident. God has a wonderful plan for your life, a plan to give you a future and a hope, to know his love and the reason why you were born. Do you think God may also have a plan for the child you are carrying?

Abortion has been an extremely popular option to terminate pregnancy in this century. But the widespread destruction of infants occurred in biblical times as well. Back in the times of Moses' and Jesus' births, the government decreed that the newly born should be killed as they came out of the mother's womb. Why?

God had a plan that a great leader, Moses, should be born. Satan clued into this and devised a plan to prevent all Israelite male children from surviving after birth. The leadership of Egypt grew afraid of how numerous and strong the Israelites were becoming and decreed that midwives were to kill all newborn males. Fortunately, the Israelite midwives decided to disobey the law and not kill the infants at birth. The mothers also resisted this practice. Otherwise, Moses would not have been spared. And if you read the story, you will see what plan God had for Moses' life and the lives of his people, who witnessed the incredible power of God among them.

God had another plan a couple of thousand years later. Jesus Christ, the Savior of all mankind, was destined to be born. During that time, King Herod was in power and decided he didn't want any competition for his throne. Hoping to kill off Jesus who was not yet a toddler, Herod issued a law saying all baby boys under two years old and living in a certain area must be killed. Warned by God, Joseph and Mary escaped with the baby Jesus. Jesus lived to fulfill God's ultimate plan of reconciling all men to God, forgiving them of their sins and welcoming them into a new family, the family of God.

So now we have our government amending laws and

Abortion: Questions to Ask Yourself

promoting abortion, the slaughter of the innocents before they are born. The law has declared that to kill a child after it is born is murder, but destroying the fetus is another matter. Or is it? Perhaps God has a plan for this generation to come to know his love and miracles in the same way he showed his love and miracles to the people of Moses' time and Jesus' time. Perhaps God has chosen your child to be a great leader. You and your child have a special place in God's heart and he wants you both to live to know him in a very special way.

If you are trying to decide whether or not to have an abortion, many people will try to give you advice and plan out your life for you. At such times you need to ask yourself, "Whose plan are they following—God's plan to give me a future and hope, or Satan's plan to destroy me?"

2. WHAT DOES A DOCTOR HAVE TO SAY ABOUT SOME OF THE PHYSICAL PROBLEMS THAT CAN BE CAUSED BY ABORTION?

Pregnancy is hard on the body no matter if the mother chooses to give birth or terminate the pregnancy. However, the aftereffects of pregnancy can be more complicated if the woman chooses to terminate the pregnancy.

Dr. Dennis Conneen is a doctor who works in an emergency room in Orange County, just south of Los Angeles. He sees the effects of abortion on women and the problems that can arise afterward. According to Dr. Conneen, "The disadvantage girls have that go to a clinic for an abortion is that clinics close at 5:00 P.M. Some girls travel to other counties to have abortions, and it's difficult for them to get help from that clinic after hours if problems arise. So those women who do have complications come in on evenings and weekends into the emergency room."

What he sees in the hospital emergency room is an eye opener for those who think they can cover up their pregnancy by having an abortion. Here are a few comments from Dr. Conneen about what he sees in the hospital on a regular basis.

"Almost every month in the Emergency Room where I work, we see a woman come in with a medical complication resulting from abortion. Out of those cases, I would say that one out of three requires hospitalization or a minor surgical procedure called a D & C. In some cases, the abortion is incomplete and there are pieces of the fetus in the uterus. These women usually experience a couple of weeks of cramping and bleeding after the abortion and decide to come in. Sometimes all they need is some blood and other fluids. Other times they need a D & C to scrape the uterus out.

"One case involved a twenty-four-year-old woman who came into the Emergency Room complaining of bleeding and cramps related to an abortion she had had one week prior. She called the doctor who performed the abortion, and he said that the abortion was complete and there should be no problems. He figured that the amount of tissue that he removed was sufficient for the age of the fetus. But sometimes, women do not give the correct conception date to the doctor who is performing the abortion. I took a look and saw the fetus's head still inside of her. The baby's head was as large as a golf ball! So I pulled it out. It was the grossest thing. You could see the trauma caused to the fetus by the abortion process. It was really beat up."

3. WHAT WILL AN ABORTION DO TO ME EMOTIONALLY?

Maybe nothing at first. The women I interviewed in this section blocked out the thoughts of the abortion as soon as they left the clinic. Later on, they began to feel guilty, and sometimes even suicidal. Many women who have had abortions don't begin to face the emotional effects until five or six years afterward. Then it suddenly dawns on them that a child could have been born and they are responsible for the decision they made.

I tend to agree with Dr. Conneen's observations about how women who have had abortions tend to behave. According to Dr. Conneen, "My own gut feeling is that many women are hardened by abortion. It's left them feeling guilty and saddened about life in a deep way. I've seen women who appear hard on the surface, noticeable by their style of language, their speech mannerisms, and the way they relate to others. There isn't a lot of softness in the way they come across."

This toughness is a sign of unresolved guilt and hurt. Only God's love and the love of other people can break through the hard exterior that says, "Don't come too close. You don't know what I've done or what's been done to me."

4. WHO WILL HELP ME IF I DON'T HAVE AN ABORTION?

Many people care about you. You just haven't met them yet. If you want to meet the ones who care about you and are willing to see you through the whole pregnancy and afterward, call one of the numbers listed below. It won't cost you a cent and your parents won't see it listed on the phone bill.

If you call and suddenly get too scared to talk or don't know what to say, then hang up. That's okay. The women answering the phone are used to people hanging up. It just means the caller is scared but really needs to talk. Just call back and say you are considering having an abortion and want to talk to someone. You will find whoever answers the phone to be really friendly and able to talk to you in such a way that you won't feel that she is a total stranger. Usually, the woman will give you another phone number to call and put you in touch with those who live close by and are able to care for you.

Lifeline	1 (800) 238-4269
National Pregnancy Hotline	1 (800) 344-7211
Birthright (U.S. & Canada)	1 (800) 328-LOVE
The Pearson Foundation (Catholic)	1 (800) 633-2252 ext. 700

PART III
Parenthood

The Parenthood Option

Listen to the voices of single mothers who never get a break from responsibilities: "Raising a child. Alone. No dad on the scene to change an occasional diaper. Where is the money for extra clothes for me? Who will watch the kid if I have a date for the movies? Where can I keep the kid while I work all day?"

Listen to their son's struggle for identity in a home devoid of a father: "I wish I had a dad. All I hear around my house is girl talk. It's rough to be a guy and live with your mom. All of her boyfriends come over and say stuff like, 'So this is the little man in your life.' Half of them don't like me. Sometimes one of her boyfriends will take me out fishing and to ball games and stuff, but just when s50liking the guy my mom breaks up with him and I don't get to see him anymore."

As you read the stories of the young women in this portion of the book, keep listening. They all had to grow up quickly, go to work, and come home to a tired, hungry, whining child. Single mothers I've talked with freely express the hardships and joys of raising their children alone. Those who marry because a baby is due or live together with their boyfriends also speak of the hardships of living with an immature dad who suddenly learns that he has to be responsible for his new family. No more partying with the guys. No more going out on the town with other girls. It's off to work and home again. No more extra spending money. Some young mothers end up having to raise two children—the newborn and the new husband or live-in boyfriend.

Raising a child in today's society takes a lot of support financially and emotionally. Out of every ten young women who become pregnant, five terminate their pregnancies by abortion, one releases her child for adoption, and four choose to become single parents. Out of the four women, one will have the support of her family. The others tough it out alone. If you are trying to decide whether to raise a child alone, ask yourself three questions:

(1) How prepared am I?
(2) How mature am I?
(3) Will my family and/or my boyfriend's family help support me financially and emotionally?

One of the girls in this section asked herself all three questions and realized that it would not be difficult for her to keep and raise her child. Through working all through high school and keeping active in sports, she had developed a greater sense of responsibility and maturity than most of her friends. In addition, her family offered to assist her as she raised her child. Her boyfriend, a longtime friend from childhood, was willing to assume the responsibility of fatherhood. And his parents also rallied to their cause and offered to assist the young couple. Everything lined up for her to become a mother. Eventually, she and her boyfriend began to live together in her mother's home. Years later, however, they still cannot afford their own place to live. And they're still not committed enough to their relationship to make it permanent.

Anybody can give birth to a child, but not everyone has what it takes to be an excellent mother. God created mothers and fathers. Both are to act as role models for children and guide them into responsible adulthood.

Think of some parents you admire. Remember when you were at a friend's house watching her mother or dad and wishing they were your parents? My best friend's mom was so cool. She spent a lot of time with us, making candy, talking, watching us swim in their pool. I wished at times that she were my mom. I spent so much time at my friend's house that her mother actually became like another mom to me. In fact, this woman and my mom were best friends, too.

I could never understand why my friends used to envy me for having such neat parents who spent a lot of time with us. They were just parents to me. I couldn't see how great they were until I saw how bad some of my other school friends had it at home.

As kids, we craved parents who would spend time with us, love us, teach us new skills, discipline us, and train us. We needed both a mom and a dad. Sometimes, we needed more than one mom and dad.

If you think of someone else's mom that you particularly like, try to identify what makes her a good mother. What kind of mom do you want to be? What kind of dad do you want your child to have? Single moms tend to hang out with other single moms, so there aren't a lot of guys around on a steady basis to act as male role models for your child. Think for a moment, whose dad do you particularly like and why? What kind of dad do you want for your child? Can your present boyfriend be that kind of a dad?

PROS AND CONS OF SINGLE MOTHERHOOD

The greatest benefit of single motherhood is knowing that your child is with you. You know how it is being raised. You get to watch it grow and can pick out what character traits are just like yours. During the first years of motherhood when you seem to be lavishing constant attention on the needs of the child, you have a sense of being needed. Eventually, the child begins to return your love. But at first it's all give and no get.

As you grow more confident in parenting, you may gain a greater sense of accomplishment in life. Finally, you feel like a somebody. You will certainly gain in maturity.

The Parenthood Option

For many young women, however, the need to work absorbs most of their time and energy, leaving little to give to a demanding infant. They are just too tired or too stressed out from money worries to enjoy their child. It's hard to raise a child when you're poor.

Some feel like their lives were cut short and begin resenting the fact that the child interrupted their plans for school or travel. They have had to put their dreams and goals on a shelf for a while until other provisions for the child fall into place.

Maybe dad will move in and marry you. But how mature is dad? Will he be sticking one bottle in the baby's mouth and another in his own? Many young mothers believe their boyfriend will marry them or another Prince Charming will ride into view and sweep mother and child away. They live in a fantasy world. Prince Charming may never come. You may be single a long, long time.

The effects of single parenting on the child will vary at different stages of the child's development. Children need two healthy role models in their life—male and female, mother and father. Moms try to be both, but it's difficult. Sons raised by single mothers long for a dad and struggle for sexual identity without a male role model. Daughters raised by single mothers also need a dad to love them and model appropriate male behavior.

If the child is left in day care for extended periods of time, he or she will be begging for your attention and be exhausted in the evenings when you want to relax after a long day at work. If you see your child only at bedtime, the child is essentially being raised without mom and dad.

A friend of mine used to work strange hours when no day-care center was open. Fortunately, her sister lived nearby and the child was of school age. At 4:00 A.M. every morning, she would dress her son and drive him over to her sister's. Once there, she would put him back to bed on the couch, and her sister would get him off to school. The boy fell asleep at school quite often.

I also know several single mothers whose children attend school all day and then are bused to a day-care center until 6:00 P.M. when their mothers pick them up on their way home from work. By that time both mother and kids are hungry and tired. When the kids are sick, mom often has to miss a day of work to stay home with them. The boss doesn't like employees missing work for the sake of kids. No day-care center accomodates sick kids. So mom stays home trying to comfort her child while she worries about missing work.

Another girl I know gave birth to a son when she was fifteen years old. She lived in her mom's house for a while trying to adjust to motherhood and waiting for her income from Aid to Families with Dependent Children, welfare, and every state and federal assistance she could obtain. Then, she moved into her own apartment. Just she and the baby. Freedom and independence at last. But her friends rarely came by to visit. How could they relate to her now that she was a mom? Eventually, a boyfriend moved in and alleviated her loneliness. She got pregnant again and decided one child was hard enough to raise so she had an abortion. The boyfriend moved out and she moved back in with her mother. She is still there, back to the same old arguments with her mother, working and raising her son.

Parenting is an incredible responsibility. If you are considering single parenting, talk to other single moms about what it's like. They'll tell you the truth. And you will begin to discover whether you can handle the job that never ends.

Waiting for Prince Charming

Pulling up in front of Cheryl's home in Los Angeles was a little intimidating even in broad daylight. A white writer in an all-black neighborhood attracts attention and suspicion. But I could tell Cheryl had already briefed her neighbors. A few young men standing further down the block stopped their conversation and stared at me as I parked the car. Cheryl was watching for me and stepped off the front porch to greet me.

Once we were inside, Cheryl introduced me to her daughter, a beautiful five-year-old. Several other children played inside, and an older youth was dispatched to watch the pack while our interview was in progress. The children marched off to another room and played quietly. Cheryl's daughter interrupted occasionally, curious about who I was.

Cheryl, a single mother who lives in southeast Los Angeles, spoke of the difficulty of raising a child alone and the longing to find a man who would step in and rescue her. Her story tells of a courageous drive to face up to responsibilities. She gave up high school dances for diapers, dates for staying at home with the baby, college scholarships for motherhood. While her family assisted her, they refused to carry the weight of responsibility and continually placed the joys of parenthood on her shoulders. Single for a period of six years, Cheryl grew up as much as her daughter and finally met that Prince Charming she was in search of years before.

Cheryl got pregnant in high school and suddenly found herself in a different world, cut off from school. "I didn't go to my prom. I didn't graduate with my class. I wasn't in my yearbook. When I look back on my years in high school I think there should have been more. I should have been there. That was my last year in school and I should have had something to show for it."

Unplanned pregnancy can ruin your whole day ... and the next ... and the next. Activities you have planned end up canceled. Who wants to attend a prom eight months pregnant? I mean, how close can you slow dance with an extended belly? When decisions arise on whether to accept a full college scholarship or to go to work to support your child, how do you choose? During the course of nine months of pregnancy, your life will change. Cheryl's old life as a high school student turned into a new life of single motherhood, and the transition was difficult.

"One day, my daughter was sick and I wanted to go out. I said, 'You guys are here. You take care of her. I'm going out.'

"My brother came over and said, 'You're not going out. Not tonight. Maybe not for a couple of years. You made this decision.'

"I couldn't resent them, really. They did so much for me, too. I just came to grips with it and dealt with the situation. For the first thirteen months after I had my baby I didn't go out and date. And I had so much life in me! So much I wanted to do!"

Cheryl didn't realize her life was going to stop. She had another life to provide for: a life that required constant attention, constant income for diapers, milk, food, and clothes, as well as medical bills that might arise. Although her family helped out with baby-sitting when she went to work and emotional support when she was frazzled, the responsibility for her daughter was hers alone. Knowing that, Cheryl rose to the challenge and decided to get as well prepared as possible before the baby arrived.

Many school districts offer alternative education for pregnant teens. Some are called "Teen Mother" or "School-age Mother" programs. They offer regular classes and provide tutoring toward obtaining the G.E.D. certificate of graduation. Classes on motherhood are also offered. Cheryl went into the program naive on all aspects of raising a child and came out well prepared for facing the next few years as a mom.

"Those classes scared me in a way," Cheryl remembered. "All the girls were pregnant at the time. We had baby dolls to learn how to change diapers and bathe them. But we also read about babies. We read about crib death and other problems. They showed us films on childbirth and that scared us. They talked about labor lasting from three to twenty-four hours. The first girl in our group to go through labor lasted eighteen hours. Eighteen hours of pain! That's the first time I wondered if I was making a mistake or if I was doing the right thing. Could I cope?"

Good question. Actually, the birth process lasts only a few hours out of a lifetime. Coping with the decision to carry a child the full nine months takes courage. But parenting takes even more courage, as well as lots and lots of patience and perseverance. You may be able to forget your schoolbooks when you run out the door, but you can't forget a baby.

"I have to thank God for the maturity and ability I had in those first months of being a mom," Cheryl said. "My older sister, the one who practically raised me, had a strong belief in God, and she was always there. When my baby was crying and I couldn't take it anymore, I would say, 'Here, will you help me?'

"And she would say, 'Okay, I'll take care of her right now, but I won't always do this for you. I didn't have this baby, you did. And you're going to take on this responsibility for yourself.'"

Fortunately, Cheryl lived with her sister and had older brothers living nearby who helped ease her into the responsibility she had chosen. Listening to an infant crying for hours because it feels sick yet doesn't have the ability to tell you where it hurts is frustrating. So frustrating, mothers end up either bursting into tears or yelling or are so wiped out that they find destructive ways to cope. If you think you can cope with being a single mother, watch yourself to see how you react when you are angry. Put yourself in a situation where you have to baby-sit a sick child overnight and see how well you deal with it. In fact, if you absolutely detest baby-sitting, what makes you think you are going to like being a twenty-four-hour parent? There are other options.

Cheryl didn't know her other options, however. "No one ever told me that if you feel like you can't cope you can give the baby up for adoption. So I felt like the only option I had was to keep her. And I couldn't see myself getting an abortion. My girlfriend's mother sat me down and talked to me for two hours. She said, 'You know, I can't see you being a mother. You have so much you want to do with your life. Why don't you do those things first and then think about becoming a mother? Get an abortion. I'll take you down to get an abortion. I'll even pay for it.' I couldn't believe it. I just couldn't have an abortion."

Lots of people are willing to give advice. Deep down inside, Cheryl knew what was right for her. If you're pregnant, you know the right decision for you to make. Your life and the life of the child growing within deserve equal consideration. God created both of you, and he promises to provide.

It took a while for Cheryl to stop dreaming about what life could be like and face reality. "Growing up, you're led to believe that some Prince Charming is going to come along and take you away. When you're from a lower income family, that's all you think about."

Her oldest brother perpetually burst her fantasy bubble. He kept telling her that she was going to make it on her own. "Don't think a man is going to want you if you're not doing that well," he reminded her. With her whole family nudging her into the challenge of making a new life for herself and the child, Cheryl started making plans for her future.

"Two months after I had her I had to go back to school. I decided that I didn't want to be on the county welfare system. This was my baby and my responsibility, so why should anybody else have to pay for her? So I went for my G.E.D. at Los Angeles City College. Classes went from 7:30 A.M. to 12:30 P.M. After class I went to work until 6:00 or 7:00 at night. I had just turned eighteen."

One of her brothers was out of work and baby-sat for Cheryl. Sometimes, the baby's father would take care of her, but he faded out of the family scene after a few months. He just wasn't interested in being a father. Nor was he interested in keeping in contact with Cheryl or the baby.

That time in Cheryl's life was one of the worst. "I hated getting up every morning—go to school, go to work, come home, take care of my baby, watch her cry in the middle of the night—and then I'd cry because I wanted her to be quiet!"

Eventually, she stopped attending school. It was getting too difficult. She took a full-time job during the day. By then, her brother worked nights and was able to keep the baby during the day. For the first two years of her child's life, Cheryl didn't have to worry about finding a baby-sitter or an infant care center. Her daughter was also able to have a male role model in her life through her uncle's influence. After a couple of years, Cheryl put her daughter in day care close to where she worked and went back to school a couple of nights a week.

One of the hardest tasks to face as a single mother is disciplining a child. No one else is around to step in and support the mom or reinforce her efforts to instill basic safety rules, obedience, manners, and values in the child. Even cute little two-year-olds can turn into monsters. Cheryl read her child development books in the teen mother program and decided to parent according to the book. "This book told me not to discipline my child—that if you talk to them they'll behave. I'll bet!" she laughed.

"I thought I had the world by the tail and knew everything. Pretty soon, though, everything started driving me crazy, and I thought I was an unfit mother. My daughter knew, at two years old, that all I was going to do was discipline her by talking to her. Pretty soon, she was talking to me like, 'You shut up. I'm not listening to you.'

"We had this glass table with crystal on it and I said to my daughter, 'Don't touch that.' I left the room, and she took that crystal and threw it. It broke all over the floor. She could have cut herself, and this book tells me not to hit her. I sat her down and talked to her for two hours. Then I cleaned up the mess and went to bed. The next morning she was on that table throwing off that crystal again."

Another incident requiring discipline occurred in the middle of a grocery store when Cheryl's daughter threw a tantrum. "I took her to the market one day and she wanted something. I said no and she fell down in the market and kicked and screamed. But that book told me I'm not supposed to hit my child. I picked her up and said, 'You don't act like that.' I was so embarrassed.

"No one can tell you how to be a mother," Cheryl continued. "Each child is different. Each mother is different. I'm not telling anyone to beat their child, but if you have a strong-willed, active child you are going to have to discipline that child faithfully. I still talk to my daughter, but I discipline her too. I spank her and put her to bed. I tell her 'yes' a lot, but it always seems like I'm telling her 'no.' :

"Raising her alone is not easy. I always have to be the

heavy. No one else is going to say, 'OK, I'll discipline her this time.' Sometimes I feel like she resents me."

Dating was another problem Cheryl encountered. Not many guys want to date a single mother. Or, if they do, they're interested only in the girl, not in the child. They're not interested in being a father, but the child of a single mother desperately longs for attention from a male role model. And then there's another pressure. As Cheryl puts it, "Guys are guys. When guys know you have a child they seem to think, 'All right, I'll take her out and show her a good time, and maybe she'll show me a good time.' They just assumed I would go to bed with them because I had been to bed with someone else."

Cheryl held out for a long time. Her brother's influence paid off. She never settled for less than the type of man who would be a good husband and father. As she began to provide for herself and her child, she developed into a different person. Gone was the immature high school student. Through successfully handling situation after situation that life threw before her path, she developed confidence and self-esteem. In time, she met her Prince Charming.

"I didn't like my fiancé at all when we met," Cheryl recalled. "We were so different. He was in college on a football scholarship, and I guess he was a big shot out there. We met at a wedding and became friends. He was so good with kids. At the time, I didn't know he was going to school to be a child psychologist."

If Cheryl had panicked and settled for any guy that came along because she was lonely or thought she couldn't cope, she could be sitting in a worse situation today. Instead, with the backing of her family, Cheryl waited and worked to meet her goals. Today, Cheryl is married to a pro football player and has another child.

Marriage? Maybe One Day

Esperanza ran with her track team one day, feeling great, no problems at home or at school. But by the next day something was seriously wrong. Was it just a bout with the flu or something greater? After staying in bed for a week, Esperanza went to the doctor for diagnosis. After all, her teammates needed her back on the track and on the softball field. What a way to let a team down—getting sick in the middle of the season. But it was not an ordinary illness. Her problem was going to grow for a period of nine months . . . and affect her for the rest of her life.

When Esperanza learned she was pregnant, she wasn't too shocked. She and her boyfriend had been going out together for a year and a half and had been sexually active for the six months before she got pregnant. She said, "I just thought, well, if it happens, it happens. We never thought about birth control. I was kind of naive about birth control. My mom never told me about the birds and the bees, so I kind of had to learn it on my own."

Some girls find themselves pregnant immediately after they lose their virginity. Other girls fool around for months before they get pregnant. In any case, unplanned pregnancy is a crisis for everyone. But a crisis does not have to be a horrendous experience. It can be an opportunity to change your life, sometimes for the better.

Any crisis situation will make you stop and think and ask yourself questions like: What do I do now? How did I get myself into this? What kind of a lifestyle do I want to live after I get through this crisis? Crises are also a time to discover your inner strengths, the stuff you are made of. They are times of difficult decisions and churning emotions. But you will live through them.

Remember that this too shall pass. It just may take a little longer than you thought.

Sometimes it helps to break a crisis down into steps. Asking yourself what to do next, then doing it, is taking that first step. Esperanza's first step was to tell her mom. For this track star, breaking the news to her mother was the biggest hurdle she had ever faced.

"It was on my mind constantly since the doctor took the blood test," Esperanza said. "Every day I wondered, 'How am I going to tell my mom? How am I going to tell my dad?'"

Family superstitions over a pending lunar eclipse finally forced Esperanza into the decision to tell her mom. Deep down, mothers often know when something is wrong, but they don't want to face the facts and sit down to figure out what is wrong. In the back of her mind, Esperanza's mom knew her daughter was pregnant. As if her mom sensed the timing was right to find out Esperanza was pregnant, the topic of the eclipse came up.

Esperanza explained how she used the eclipse to tell her mother of her pregnancy. "My mom's side of the family was superstitious and followed the signs of the eclipses and all of that. I remember my grandmother telling me that when women are pregnant during a time of an eclipse they should tie a bunch of keys or paper clips together like a chain and put it around their stomach to protect the baby. They say an eclipse takes away something from the baby like a finger or a toe or creates a hairlip. I was going to be four months pregnant when an eclipse was due, and I didn't want anything to happen to my baby. I didn't know what to do. I had to tell my mom so she could tell me what I was supposed to do.

"Just when I got my nerve up to tell her, my mom brought up the story and said she needed to call my aunt, who was pregnant at the time, and remind her to put the key belt around her. I said, 'Oh, really?'

"Then she said, 'Can you think of anybody else we need to tell?'

"I said, 'Well mom, better start pulling out the keys.' She had no idea about me. She looked at me and her face dropped. She said, 'What do you mean?'

"I said, 'Well mom, I'm pregnant.'

"She didn't talk to me. She just got up and started looking through the drawers for all the keys and paper clips she could find and started putting them on me. She didn't say anything to me all that night, but then the next morning she said, 'How are we going to tell your dad?'"

Esperanza left it up to her mother to decide how to break the news to her father, who had quite a gruff way about him. He wasn't a mean dad; he was just a man of few words. No one really knew where he stood on things or what he thought. He sat around and grunted a lot rather than talking.

Esperanza's mother started calling her father "grandpa." "Grandpa! Grandpa Fred!" she said, "You're going to be a grandpa."

He didn't take the news very well at first. Several times Esperanza caught him watching her, but he didn't say anything. But pretty soon, he started babying her and showing her that he cared. It took him about a week before he could talk to Esperanza, and then he said, "It better be a boy." Fortunately for grandpa, she had a boy.

It takes a while for parents to get past the shock of realizing that their daughter, their little girl, is going to have a baby. If you are still in high school, they haven't quite finished raising you. They think you can't be a parent because you aren't finished being parented yet. After getting over the shock, they start feeling sad for you. All of the things they wanted for you, all of the dreams they had for you, are instantly changed. They know how difficult it is to raise a family and provide for a child. Knowing you as well as they do, they also realize how difficult it will be for you to raise a child.

Next your parents will start to blame themselves. Thinking they failed as parents, they lash out in anger. In a crisis, parents feel as much pain as their child. They may react violently to the news of your pregnancy, but they are just expressing the hurt that they feel. Usually they will calm down and be a great support to you.

As soon as she found out she was pregnant, Esperanza told her boyfriend. Telling Eddie was easier than telling her parents. She knew Eddie well. Her dad's family and Eddie's family lived in the same neighborhood, so she had known Eddie as a child. When he was about fifteen, he started noticing Esperanza as something more than a childhood buddy. When she turned seventeen, he asked her on a date. Esperanza turned him down.

"I said, 'No, I don't want to go out with you. You have too many girlfriends. You're probably dating somebody right now.' He said, 'No I'm not. What about you? I see all these boys hanging around you.' He kept on begging me, so finally I said I'd go out with him. He got my phone number and called me the very next day. We stayed on the phone chatting and chatting. Then he said maybe he'd call me tomorrow. He called me every single day. Maybe the second or third week after we had gone out on the date he asked me if I wanted to be his girlfriend."

When Esperanza called Eddie and told him about the pregnancy, she could tell that he didn't know what to think of the situation. Immediate visions of being murdered by her father flooded his mind. He came over that night and said, "How are we going to tell your dad?" They kept it a secret for a while.

After her family found out, she invited Eddie over, pretending that the news still hadn't been broken. He walked into the house and said, "Hi Fred" and pretended like nothing was different, that there was nothing to hide. Just watching Eddie try to act so normal sent Esperanza into hysterical laughter. Finally, she took Eddie aside and told him that her parents knew. He was embarrassed to go back into the living room and face them. But it was too late. He was in the house.

"I said, 'Look, did they beat you up or bite your head off? Don't worry about it.' He was nervous about my dad's reaction, but my dad really liked Eddie. After all, he watched Eddie grow up. His dad used to take him everywhere, so when the guys would hang out, there was little Eddie running around. There was no way he would hurt Eddie or get really angry."

Now that her family and Eddie's family were informed of the pregnancy, Esperanza had several more hurdles to face. She decided to quit school and handled that hurdle. But she needed to keep earning extra income. Esperanza's next step was to tell her boss and see if she could keep working throughout her pregnancy. She worked at a children's after-school center creating activities that would keep the children occupied until their mothers came for them. Most of the mothers were single parents, so Esperanza knew firsthand of their difficulties. When she told her boss, she said it wouldn't be a problem. She continued working through her whole pregnancy.

Pregnancy is a condition most people notice right away, especially as the months pass. Some women feel very self-conscious, and to some women the most difficult part of being pregnant is being stared at on the street, at church, anywhere in public. People seem to take special notice of pregnant women.

Friends began to notice Esperanza at Mass. "I remember going to church while I was pregnant, and I felt like everyone was staring at me. I was kind of embarrassed running into old schoolmates. They would say, 'Look at you. You're going to have a baby.' But nobody ever said anything to put me down. As a matter of fact, our priest came and blessed Andrew the day he was born."

Now that they had a child to consider, it was time to decide how they would have the baby and where they would live. They ruled out marriage. Abortion or adoption were not even options. They were excited about having a child.

"Eddie and I talked about living together," Esperanza said. "There were no negative comments from him about not being able to handle the relationship or responsibilities of fatherhood. I was pretty mature. I knew my own mind and was pretty stable. I think we were both ready to handle it. We both came from really supportive families, too. That helped. Some Hispanic families are very cold. I know some Catholic Hispanic families who would have kicked their daughter out for being pregnant before marriage. We aren't a huggy, kissy family, yet we're really close when trouble or something comes up."

Esperanza was very fortunate to have as much family support as she did. This is rare. Rarer still is having a boyfriend who is willing to go through the entire experience with you. Despite all the support, however, Esperanza still wasn't in the ideal situation. Even though Eddie was ready to rise to the challenge of parenthood, he wasn't financially ready. Nor was he ready to marry Esperanza.

They decided to live with her parents. Eddie's parents were willing to take them in, but they lacked the extra room. Esperanza's mother threw a baby shower. Then all they had to do was save enough money for the birth expenses.

Esperanza had a long talk with her parents about how she would have the baby. "We had to decide whether to go with a midwife or a hospital. I wanted to have it at home because I had an aunt who had twins at home. Eddie was a little nervous about the idea, but we decided to save on the hospital bill. We signed up for natural childbirth classes, and the instructor gave me the number of a midwife. The total cost for checkups and delivery was about $800."

These days you can't deliver a baby that inexpensively. The cost of delivering a child is rising as lawsuits increase. Midwives need to be licensed and must work in close alliance with a physician. And if you can find a midwife, she will probably be expensive. Doctors and hospitals do cost a great deal, but special birthing rooms in hospitals allow the mother to return home shortly after giving birth. This cuts down on the hospital bill.

Another concern is insurance. Without insurance, it is difficult to find a doctor willing to deliver a child. A number of doctors are unwilling to take patients on government assistance because it ends up costing the doctor more in malpractice insurance than he would earn from delivering the child.

Finally, unforeseen complications can cause the bill to increase dramatically. What you thought would cost only $2,500 for the delivery could turn into a $10,000 problem. Clearly, financing the delivery can be as difficult as raising the child afterward.

Esperanza was well prepared for the birth process. She and Eddie knew what was going to occur during labor, and regular checkups kept them informed of the baby's health.

Esperanza's labor and delivery were extraordinarily easy. "I pushed maybe three times and Andrew came out," she said. "I was in labor only three hours."

Mother and child came home, and Eddie moved in a week later. They began to settle into family life. Pretty soon, it was time for Esperanza to return to work. They needed the money.

During the first two years, she worked part time while

her mother took care of Andrew. After that, he was old enough for Esperanza to take to work. Fortunately, the club allowed employees to bring their children without charging them the regular fees. Now that her son is older, he attends a Head Start school program. This special program enables lower income, minority children to gain a head start in education. The school also takes care of Andrew's medical and dental appointments.

"That really helped because we didn't have any medical insurance. Andrew never had any physical problems, but without insurance we would have been wiped out financially if anything ever happened."

Because Esperanza was technically a single mother, she was eligible for government assistance, but she and Eddie provided for their own needs without applying for aid. They managed fairly well. Still, they have their moments of adjusting to parenthood. Esperanza said, "You go from school, where you have no bills and keep all your money, and suddenly you have to pay rent and pour your money into milk and diapers. You have bills to pay and extra food to buy. You get to the point where it's no longer you. You have responsibility for someone else now. And Andrew was my first responsibility. I had to mature pretty fast."

As if the financial burdens weren't enough to cope with, Eddie needed to learn how to deal with a child. Esperanza was already used to raising children, having been prepared by working at the children's club and talking with other single mothers. But for Eddie being a father was difficult at first.

"It took Eddie a while to grow into being a dad," Esperanza remembered. "When Andrew first started walking he would say, 'No, no, no, don't touch this. No, no, no ...' and slap his hands. But after a while he learned that to discipline him you don't need to hit him. You can just distract his attention and give him something else to play with. Andrew was into everything. One day he threw baby powder all over the room. I laughed. But when Eddie walked into the room he was really upset. I said, 'Hey, mellow out. He's only a baby. He doesn't know what he's doing.' It took him a long time to relax around Andrew and get into the father role. He's doing all right now that Andrew understands that no means no. Eddie feels a lot more like the boss now. It makes him feel good to be in authority."

Now it sounds like everything is going great for the young family. Esperanza is still working at the children's club and, at $7 an hour, is earning twice the salary she started at. Without a high school diploma or other job training, it is difficult to earn better money. Andrew is doing well at school. Eddie is going for his contractor's license and earning enough to keep food on the table. And Esperanza's parents are still willing to let them all live under their roof while they pay the majority of the rent. It seems that things couldn't be any better. However, there is always someone ready to stir up the nest. In Esperanza's case, her dad's godfather was living in a trailer parked in their yard, and he had a few things to say about the situation.

"So, when are you and Eddie going to get married?" he would ask. Every Sunday after Mass he would say to Esperanza, "I think it's about time you and honeybunch thought about getting married. You've got a child and you're living in sin, so . . ."

Esperanza said to me, "I still don't know why we're not married. I'm ready at any time, but I guess Eddie still isn't ready. After I had Andrew I would bring it up and Eddie would tell me, 'When the time is right, we'll get married. When I get married, I want to have a big wedding with lots of people and lots of food and beer and we'll be paying for it ourselves.' I figure when Eddie gets into his thirties and matures a little more and gets some money ahead, he'll say, 'The time is right.'"

Esperanza was in a fortunate position when she got pregnant: she had total family support, and her boyfriend was also willing to take an active father role and support his new family. More mature than her peers, she rose to the challenge of parenting with the same psychological determination that caused her to excel in sports.

Despite all the support, however, Esperanza still faces the difficulty of trying to create a family while her boyfriend eludes the ties of marriage. She is frustrated over how long it is taking for her boyfriend to gain enough experience to earn a substantial living and mature as a father. Their son is now five years old, and they still live with her parents.

If a man isn't willing to marry, to form an unbreakable bond with a woman he professes to love and care for, then something is lacking. Esperanza sensed that as she spoke. How much do you think Eddie really loves her if he wants to leave the option open to walk out any time he wants to? The chances are that if they have been together for the last seven years, they will probably stay together. Or will they?

Single parenting is hard, but so is living with someone who is not committed to you.

Searching for Love

Are you looking for love in all the wrong places? If someone had asked Kay that question sooner, she might have taken a long look at what she was headed into. It took a few years for Kay to find the love she was searching for. By then, she had become pregnant twice. The first time she ended the pregnancy by abortion. The second time, she met the overwhelming compassion and love of Jesus Christ and decided to keep her child. Through it all, she learned that true love never fails, keeps no records of wrongs, and always protects, trusts, and perseveres. Through it all, she met a higher love.

Even cheerleaders get the blues. High school days are not always happy days. While Kay was in high school, her family life changed abruptly. Her older brothers and sisters moved out on their own. Her mother died, and within six months her father moved his new wife into the house. Kay suddenly felt alone in a house no longer hers.

"My stepmom wouldn't let me bring my dates home," Kay recalled. "She had no trust in me. She accused me of sleeping around and always said I would get pregnant. I was a cheerleader in high school and somebody made up this rumor that I was sleeping with all of the football players. My stepmom heard the rumor but never talked to me about it; she just assumed it was true and told my dad. So I thought that if my parents didn't trust me and my dad already thought I had slept with the whole football team, why was I still trying to stay a virgin?"

Rumors are vicious. They start as easily as striking a match and catch fire as they spread throughout the community. Pretty soon, everyone who hears the rumor gets burnt, their perceptions become warped, and they begin to shut themselves off from hearing or seeing the truth. But the one who bears the brunt of the rumor can be charred beyond recognition. In Kay's case, the rumor about her led her to act it out. Rather than confronting the situation, she allowed herself to get burnt.

Kay started "going parking," as they called it in Texas. "I went from being a prude to coming on to my boyfriend's best friend. My boyfriend already knew I wouldn't sleep with him and respected that, so I went out with his best friend."

Meanwhile, a group of Quakers moved into town and started witnessing in the community. Kay began to attend one of their high school Bible studies. "My real mom was a Christian and taught me all of my morals and values before she died, so I was walking around feeling miserable that I had compromised. I knew the sex thing was a big issue and started doing my own Bible study on fornication. I knew it was wrong, that it was a sin, but I didn't know the consequences of it would affect me for the rest of my life. I didn't know that there is a blessing in sex, that God created it to be fun between a man and his wife and disastrous between those who aren't man and wife."

Like all of us, Kay knew the truth about the hurt she was walking into and was beginning to understand that God loved her enough to warn her about the problems that result from sin. Yet she still pursued a deeper relationship with her boyfriend Jack. She was looking for love, for a way out of the situation at home, and she thought her boyfriend was the key. But the key was already in her hand. Someone was knocking at the door of her heart, longing for her to turn the key and let him in so that he could give her all the love she longed for.

Jesus stood by, softly knocking. He called to Kay and offered her a new life. All she had to do was say, "Come into my life, Lord Jesus. I've made a mess of things and fallen into sin. Please forgive me and help me to start over." And Jesus would have begun to help her deal with all the emotional situations at home and at school. Jesus would have dealt with the rumors and helped her remain strong at home. Jesus would have given a new direction to her life and filled her with his love. But Kay had other plans—her own.

"I felt like my parents wanted me to move out," Kay said. "They kept saying, 'You're going to move out when you're eighteen,' so I thought they wanted me out. They had put so many restrictions on my life because of the rumors that I couldn't breathe. So I manipulated Jack's parents into letting me move into their spare bedroom."

After a while, Jack and Kay started sneaking back and forth into each others' rooms at night. Rising before his parents discovered their affair, they would sneak back into their own rooms in the morning. It took a while for his parents to catch on. When Kay went to work for Jack's dad, he finally told her that if she was going to live in his house, she was going to have to stay in her own room.

By then, Jack had gone off to college, and Kay decided to move into her brother's house. Every week, Kay would decide not to compromise her Christian values anymore and determine not to sleep with Jack. Every weekend, Jack came home from college, and because their relationship was based on sex, they would give in to their desires. Kay thought she was in love with him. By Christmas, she discovered that she was pregnant.

"I used birth control pills but got pregnant anyway. Sometimes I would forget to take a pill and go back on them later. I kept thinking that I wasn't going to have sex anymore so I would stop taking them for a week or so. Then Jack would come home and I'd pull out the birth control pills."

Kay might as well not have taken any pill at all as take them so irregularly. Birth control pills must be taken every day in order to stop the ovulation process and prevent pregnancy. Missing just one pill can start the ovulation process and allow a woman to become pregnant. Stop taking the pill and your chances of becoming more fertile increase.

Kay tried to stop having sex with Jack by not taking her pills. But it is almost impossible to stop having sex with someone if it is a secret relationship. If Kay had let the secret out to someone she trusted, that person could have stood by to help her break off the relationship. If you are in a situation that is out of control, find help. Talking about the situation, confessing it to someone, takes away the powerful grip it has on you. Secrets are like handcuffs that chain you to the bed. Someone needs to help you take them off.

Kay told Jack that she was pregnant, and Jack convinced himself that it wasn't true. He didn't want to face up to the situation. Kay said, "I thought I would keep the baby, but Jack wouldn't acknowledge that I was even pregnant. So my brother and a few others helped me to pay for an abortion. The day I went in, I had this fantasy that Jack would find out where I was and call the clinic and ask me not to do it. After the abortion I lost fifty percent of what I felt for him. How could he love me and let his baby be killed? Then it dawned on me. How could he love me if he didn't even love God?"

Kay was still attending Bible studies, but Jack had no interest in God. His parents were Christians and often invited the two of them to church. They never went. But now, in the midst of her pain, Kay began to realize that only God could give her the love that she needed.

"The day after the abortion, Jack was Mr. Charm. He acted like, 'Let's forget the whole thing.' I couldn't stand him, but I had met all sorts of other guys with a lot more problems and thought at least I knew what Jack was like. At least I was safe with him. We had a bundle of troubles, but at least I knew what they were."

They continued on in their relationship. Kay worked while Jack studied in a nearby college. Eventually rumors started getting back to her that Jack was dating other girls and sleeping around. It didn't surprise her. Kay still held on to her relationship with him. Eventually, she sensed that she was pregnant again. She had thought that if the pill didn't work the first time, she would just go off of it. Whatever happened, happened. And happen it did.

Although it wasn't confirmed, Kay knew that she was pregnant. She wanted out of the situation but chose to deny that she had a problem that wouldn't go away. She was stuck.

One of her brothers went into a six-week Christian discipleship program called Agape Force and came out of the program a changed man. He was off drugs and deeply committed to a relationship with God. Kay decided she needed that kind of change and entered the program still denying her pregnancy.

"The first week I was there I kept praying, 'Please God, don't let me be pregnant.' They spent the whole week discussing dating and relationships. I cried all week. One of the speakers got up and said, 'Some girls think they can pray "Oh God, don't let me be pregnant," but they don't realize that if you go from point A to point B, you're going to end up with the repercussions of that action.' That hit home."

Part way into the program, Kay's counselor sensed why Kay was so emotional and asked her if she thought she was pregnant. Kay said yes. A doctor added his confirmation. And Kay was left with a decision. Her counselor asked her what she was going to do.

"In those three weeks in the program I had discovered how much God loved me. I always felt worthless until I found out how much my heavenly Father valued me. And then I realized that God felt the same about this baby as he did me. My focus changed from 'What am I going to do? How can I raise this child on my own?' to 'God will take care of this child.'"

Kay decided to keep the child. She knew Jack would want to marry her and wrote him a letter breaking off the relationship. For a couple of months afterward, he pressured her to marry him. By then, Kay had returned to church in her hometown. The pastor's wife found out about Kay's pregnancy and gently asked her if she would like to give a testimony in church of how God worked in her life during her time in the Agape Force program. Kay stood up in church and told them how she had discovered the love of God. And then she broke down, sobbing out her story of being pregnant. The pastor's wife stood up and asked the church to rally to Kay's support, and she also committed herself to helping Kay all the way through this pregnancy. The church's response was overwhelmingly positive.

"Through the whole thing, they loved me and nurtured me, showing me I was forgiven. They even paid the whole bill and gave me a shower. At first, I thought they were all nerds, but the love of God that they expressed won me over. I started getting really committed to God," Kay said.

For months, she struggled with loneliness and desperately wanted a husband, someone who would be a father to her child. Yet she didn't date anyone. She left it up to God. "I prayed that God would show my pastor who I was going to marry because I didn't trust myself. I always picked jerks, guys who wouldn't be good for me." Three months after her daughter was born, her pastor realized that a young man he knew from another town should meet Kay. He called him and invited him over. It was love at first sight. Kay knew inside that this was the right man for her. And he felt the same. Within a few months they were married.

As soon as Kay decided to let go of the way she had decided to live life, she took her key and opened up the door to her heart. And Jesus came in with all of his love. He brought her into a whole different family called the family of God, the church. Pretty soon, she had more mothers and fathers and brothers and sisters than she knew what to do with. As she began to get to know them, she realized that they weren't "nerds." They were just like her . . . people learning to receive God's love and give it back to others.

Kay wasn't a single mother for long, but many single mothers find themselves living alone for years, trying to quench their loneliness with a string of messed-up relationships. Kay was able to learn to love only after she received the love of God. Single mother or not, searching for love in all the wrong places leads only to a life of pain. But the good news is that love is as close as opening up the door of your heart and asking Jesus, the giver of perfect love, to come in and change your life. Jesus is standing there knocking right now. Even as you read this a little chill is going through you. That is the breeze of the Lord beginning to come into the door of your heart. Open it all the way and welcome him. You'll discover another love.

Parenting: Where to Turn from Here

1. ASK GOD WHAT HIS PERFECT WILL FOR YOU IS IN THIS SITUATION.

God knows you are pregnant. He is the one who started the procreative processes at work in you, determining the sex, size, and all the unique features of your child as it grows in your womb. He has a plan for every life and will tell you what he plans for you and this baby.

If you attend a church, make an appointment with your pastor and see what help the church might give you. Most local churches have a few women who are very loving and willing to help out. They are part of God's plan to help you.

If you decide to become a single parent, God will be right there for you. He has a special place in his heart for single mothers and fatherless children.

The Bible refers to single mothers as "widows," women who do not have husbands. The word *orphans* in the Bible is often translated as "the fatherless," those who do not have a father, whether they are children or adults without a living father. God is a Father to all who ask him into their lives. He says so in Psalm 68:5: "A father to the fatherless, a defender of widows, is God in his holy dwelling." And he says it a different way in Psalm 10:14—"But you, O God, do see trouble and grief; you consider it to take it in hand. The victim commits himself to you; you are the helper of the fatherless."

God promises that he will provide and commands his people, the church, to assist in providing for single mothers and children. Unfortunately, some people in churches do not think they have any responsibility to help out single mothers. But God says they do. Part of a person's income is to be given to the local church. This money is called a tithe, and it is used to provide a living for the clergy as well as to help needy people, including the fatherless and the widows. Those who consider themselves religious are not to gossip about pregnant girls. The true believers, the best of Christians, will "look after orphans and widows in their distress and . . . keep [themselves] from being polluted by the world" (James 1:27).

2. CALL ONE OF THE COUNSELORS WHO ARE AVAILABLE TO HELP PREGNANT TEENS.

Pregnancy counselors will not force you into any decision. They are there to help you with what you want to do. If you need housing while you are pregnant and for a while afterwards to give you and the baby time to start a new life together, they will help. Many crisis pregnancy centers have special housing available for those who cannot live at home during their pregnancy or find that their parents are too hostile towards them. The pregnancy counselors will be there for you all during your pregnancy and will help you make arrangements for support after the baby comes.

Lifeline	1 (800) 238-4269
National Pregnancy Hotline	1 (800) 344-7211
Birthright (U.S. & Canada)	1 (800) 328-LOVE
The Pearson Foundation (Catholic)	1 (800) 633-2252 ext. 700

3. TALK TO YOUR MOTHER ABOUT YOUR DECISION TO BECOME A PARENT. FIND OUT HOW MUCH SUPPORT YOU CAN EXPECT FROM HER AND YOUR FATHER.

Talking to your mother about your pregnancy may be difficult. But most mothers want to talk to their daughters, and your mother should be the first place you turn to for help. You need to find out if she will help you and whether you can live at home with your baby for a few years until you get your life on course.

By the time you get through with this conversation, you will know where you stand. If your parents offer no support, don't be discouraged. If you want to raise your baby, other assistance is available.

4. GET READY FOR THE BIRTH AND PARENTHOOD.

Consider taking natural childbirth classes such as Lamaze. Then think about other ways to prepare: tour the hospital, throw a baby shower, attend parenting classes, get counseling, and talk to other single moms.

Read books about childbirth and parenting. One excellent book to consider is *The Handbook for Pregnant Teenagers* written by Linda Roggow and Carolyn Owens and published by Zondervan. It is available in your local Christian bookstore. While you're in the store, pick up a few other titles that catch your eye. Reading is a great way to gain more information and prepare yourself for the days to come.

5. FINISH YOUR HIGH SCHOOL EDUCATION.

Many school districts offer a teen mother program where you attend classes with other pregnant girls at a different location than your regular high school. Education classes are interspersed with classes on parenting. Teen mother programs prepare you for everything from the birth process itself to changing diapers and caring for sick infants. Ask your school counselor about a teen mother program if she hasn't already suggested one.

Attending classes towards your G.E.D. at night is also an option if you do not want to attend school pregnant or enroll in a special teen mother program. Finishing high school is usually a prerequisite to obtaining a decent job. Working at McDonald's just won't pay enough to support you and a child.

6. TALK TO YOUR BOYFRIEND AND SEE HOW MUCH HE PLANS TO BE IN THE PICTURE WHEN THE CHILD IS BORN.

Before you talk to him, it helps to have a list of questions available so you can keep him on the topic of conversation. Writing down questions ahead of time keeps you both from avoiding the issue of parenthood.

Write down questions about marriage. If he is only willing to live with you, then he doesn't care enough about you to form an unbreakable bond. Write down questions about visiting rights and child support payments if he wants to take an active father role. If he is in the U.S. Armed Forces, child support payments will be taken directly out of his paycheck whether he likes it or not.

Consult with counselors at a crisis pregnancy clinic or look up Legal Aid in your local phone book for advice on visiting rights and child support payments.

If you and your boyfriend plan to get married, have him ask his parents how much they will assist in the support and care of his new family until he gets on his feet financially.

7. MAKE GOD A PART OF YOUR PARENTING.

If you think parenting is overwhelming, you're right. Most older, married couples plan for quite a while before they decide to have children. But just remember to take life one day at a time. Each day brings new surprises and new energy. And God stands by, waiting for you to talk to him. He can show you how to parent. Ask him to point out the way.